"Wow. This is an amazing book. I firmly believe that most of what ails us affects us physically, emotionally and spiritually. We're fearfully and wonderfully made. And that's why the healing process is often more involved than we'd like it to be. Yet it's the path to true, sustainable freedom. In her trademark way, Laura offers hard-fought biblical wisdom and disciplined research that equip and empower us to get well, live free and embrace the wholeness that Jesus won for us. If you're ready to move beyond symptom management to a place that calls for faith, hope and a little bit of discipline, you may just find the healing you've longed for all along. I'll be praying for you."

Susie Larson, national speaker; show host; author, *Fully Alive: Learning to Flourish, Mind, Body, and Spirit*"

"As a nutritionist helping people for two decades, I can attest to these truths. I've grieved the ignorance among the medical community about the spiritual, and the ignorance among the faith community about the medical. Read this and find answers along with practical steps you can take today!"

Elizabeth Reed, M.S.N.

"Laura Harris Smith is an anointed Kingdom leader. She has discovered some astonishing principles unleashed in these writings that, when received by faith and with a heart of worship to our God, will help bring natural and supernatural renewal to your body, mind and spirit."

Jeff Deyo, worship leader; professor; author, *Awakening Pure Worship: Cultivating a Closer Friendship with God*

"I believe Laura's new book, *Get Well Soon*, will have a tremendous impact on the way people understand God'- on divine health and healing. For too teaching have 'clouded' the thinki

from living their lives to the fullest. This book is a tool and treasure map to help bring you into the light of neglected truth."

Franco Gennaro, CEO, Family First Health;
patent holder, Flu-B-Gone and Immune Booster Express;
author, *The Coming Global Flu Crisis: Fact or Fiction*

"Laura Harris Smith offers a practical and attainable guide to seeking natural and supernatural healing both internally and externally. This book will transform your life!"

Ty and Charlene Bollinger, founders,
The Truth About Cancer

GET WELL SOON

GET WELL SOON

Natural and Supernatural Remedies
for Vibrant Health

LAURA HARRIS SMITH,

C.N.C., M.S.O.M.

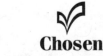

Chosen

a division of Baker Publishing Group
Minneapolis, Minnesota

© 2019 by Laura H. Smith

Published by Chosen Books
11400 Hampshire Avenue South
Bloomington, Minnesota 55438
www.chosenbooks.com

Chosen Books is a division of
Baker Publishing Group, Grand Rapids, Michigan

Printed in the United States of America

Library of Congress Cataloging-in-Publication Data

Names: Smith, Laura Harris, author.
Title: Get well soon : natural and supernatural remedies for vibrant health / Laura Harris Smith, C.N.C., M.S.O.M.
Description: Minneapolis, Minnesota : Chosen, a division of Baker Publishing Group, [2019] | Includes bibliographical references and index.
Identifiers: LCCN 2018042311| ISBN 9780800799175 (pbk.) | ISBN 9781493417407 (e-book)
Subjects: LCSH: Health. | Health—Psychological aspects. | Health—Religious aspects. | Health attitudes. | Mind and body.
Classification: LCC RA776.5 .S579 2019 | DDC 613—dc23
LC record available at https://lccn.loc.gov/2018042311

The information given in Get Well Soon is biblical, pastoral and spiritual in nature. It is not professional counsel and should not be viewed as such. Laura Harris Smith, Chosen Books and Baker Publishing Group specifically disclaim all responsibility for any liability, loss or risk, personal or otherwise, that is incurred as a consequence, directly or indirectly, of the use of and/or application of any contents of this book.

Cover design by Emily Weigel

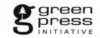

For Pop.

Thank you for raising, influencing,
inspiring, forgiving, loving . . .
and remembering me.

I'll always be your girl.

Contents

Part Three
Get Well, Stay Well

Foreword

Too many people are experiencing the frustrations of sickness and suffering. The search for a better sense of conscious well-being and relief from debilitating illnesses is intense!

To be a responsible steward of our bodies is to understand how the body works, along with understanding the vital role personal responsibility plays in our health-and-wellness experience. When sickness comes, it is essential that we employ time-honored principles that will, in cooperation with both natural and spiritual laws, build up and restore the whole person—*body, mind and spirit*.

Laura Harris Smith has given us in these pages a very clear, simple, instructive and empowering road map for providing hope to the despondent, health to the sick and rest for the weary. Her own significant health challenges, intense research, health education and spiritual walk are a powerful witness to the "get well soon" theme of this book that I believe you as the reader will find both inspirational and empowering. As she shows us how she and others use these powerful health principles that she talks about, we develop a vicarious connection to her special gift of caring and sharing, which is a vital part of her multifaceted background as a gifted communicator, TV host, health educator, church founder and pastor. You will be both encouraged by and convinced of the power of the biblically based principles she conveys.

Part one of *Get Well Soon* shows us how to integrate body, mind and spirit harmoniously for maintaining and restoring health and vitality in this increasingly sick-ravaged world. It starts by having us boldly and assertively confront our state of health and render explicit how well we really want to be. It shows the importance of taking full responsibility for our health, doing all that we can, and then reinforcing our efforts with a right relationship with God. God supplies the "divine supplement" to the full spectrum of human efforts that are in harmony with His time-honored natural health laws.

Laura convincingly asserts and helps us understand that God's will and purpose for us is to thrive, and not just survive, on this planet. God is not responsible for illnesses. When we are in harmony with His designed purpose for us, however, it places us on the road to outrageous health and vitality. We are reminded that God always has and always will have our highest health and happiness in His will. When we unite with Him through His natural laws of health, with a sincere, humble and prayerful attitude, we are equipped and empowered to do everything He has purposely designed us for. He is the Father of Lights, and our light becomes the designed reflection of His divine Light.

Laura validates her assertions with sound biblical passages that help us bathe in the richness of the blessings God has for us to reverse any personal or generational curses we may be experiencing. Using the Word of God as the unequivocal foundation for all the power and majesty of the universe, she helps us understand the importance of our thoughts and words in experiencing true health and wellness. She guides us through the power and proper practice of prayer, understanding the role that miracles and healings play in overcoming any and all *known* and *unknown* diseases—physically, mentally and spiritually.

When you read this book, you will develop a richer appreciation of God's love and personal involvement in all aspects of your well-being. Laura eloquently presents Him in the full character of both His *spiritual* and *natural* laws, which are the foundational elements of the most powerful system known to man for preventing and reversing all named and unnamed health issues. He is not an impersonal God, but a God who provides fellowship with us through His Word. When we pray to Him, He provides a path to health for us, either by direct miracles or by natural healing pathways. Laura also helps us understand and differentiate between those two. God is always working for the good of those who love Him, and He will not turn away from those who choose to return to Him. She ends part one by encouraging you to love the new you that is developed from a prayerful practice of the concepts and principles she has covered, with the following encouraging shout-out: Keep an eternal perspective! Keep an eternal perspective!

In part two of *Get Well Soon*, you will experience a rich and empowering series of prayers for the 15 body systems. These healing prayers cover over 200 compromised health conditions. Laura blends an empowering knowledge of anatomy and physiology with the mechanisms of the disease processes and with powerful prayers for cementing what you learned in part one. Each of the 15 body systems is reinforced with a powerful declaration, a personal blessing, an "A-list" of do's and don'ts for that system (what to *Avoid, Add, Allow, Apply, Anoint* and *Ask*), practical meal suggestions and encouraging testimonies.

Laura Harris Smith is going to provide you with a clear picture of how to *get well soon*. I can assure you that if you take heed to the words in this book, they can transform your life and provide you with greater health and vitality, with the bonus of a closer walk with God.

I have read this book. It makes sense; it is not complicated. It is not authoritarian, but it gives you the support you need to make a difference. As I have seen so often in my practice, when you incorporate the principles in these pages (even though this is not always easy), there will be a positive difference in your health, vitality, life and longevity, *temporally* and *eternally*.

May you continue to receive God's richest blessings as Laura takes you on this blessed journey to help you pursue your physical, mental and spiritual walk with the one and only Master Healer!

Jim Sharps, N.D., H.D., Dr.N.Sc., Ph.D., president and CEO, International Institute of Original Medicine

Acknowledgments

Thank you, Jennifer Callaway, R.N., for being the first set of expert eyes on the 200-plus medically detailed healing prayers, as well as for alphabetizing and cross-referencing the infirmity index. The way you love and care for your patients as a nurse has always impressed me, but now the way you have loved and cared for my readers has made me love you all the more. You have made it easier for them to find their healing prayer quickly inside these pages, so on behalf of all of them and from the bottom of my heart, thank you.

And many thanks to you, Dr. Jim Sharps, for lending your name to the cover, for writing the foreword, for double-checking my facts inside, and for offering your enthusiasm to the entire project. And of course, I cannot fail to thank you for founding the school that changed my life and equipped me for the road I am on—the International Institute of Original Medicine. You and Dr. Elisa are both rising and shining stars in the field of body, mind and spirit health, and I am indebted to you both for your godly guidance and care.

Part One

Employing Your Spirit and Mind for Bodily Healings

You have a life to live! Are you ready to live it? Imagine the healthiest, happiest version of yourself, and let's go find you. No matter what condition you are in today, get ready to take some steps toward understanding how to gain and maintain total body, mind and spirit health. God has a tailor-made strategy to help you walk in wholeness, and my goal is to come alongside you in the process and help you find it. I believe that as you take the steps I outline in the pages ahead and pray the body system blessings and healing prayers, you will find all the health and strength you need to live out the days God has planned for you in the earth and to accomplish all the things He has for you to do.

As you work through this book, you will see various online resources I have prepared for you. I hope you will take advantage of them. For example, there will be opportunities to take notes or even make timelines that will help correlate your physical symptoms to important life passages or emotional events. So for convenience, I have created downloadable forms to help you with this process each time. You can either visit the URLs as they are offered to you, or you can go ahead of time to lauraharrissmith.com/forms and download them now. It may help you to have copies of each form so you can write on them freely as you take inventory of your current health, investigate the root causes of any conditions that are afflicting you, and create a timeline that tracks the history of those conditions. You can keep these sheets handy for future reference, too, since they will soon become a testimony of how far the Lord has taken you on your path to wholeness.

Then, as you will see when you reach part two, you can also visit lauraharrissmith.com/blessings to hear me speak each body system blessing over you via video. I made fifteen of these videos and look forward to connecting with you in each one. Also, since space is limited, as I outline health-giving foods for every body system, you can also find some expanded recipes at lauraharrissmith.com/recipes, not to mention some compelling testimonies of people who used food as medicine at lauraharris smith.com/testimonies. And finally, before, during and after your completion of this book, you can keep up with my free offers and giveaways that have to do with body, mind and spirit health by liking my author page on Facebook at facebook.com/LauraHarrisSmithPage/. Let me hear from you as you find healing in the pages of this book—body, mind or spirit—so that I can include your breakthrough story on our testimony page.

1

Decide How Well
You Really Want to Be

So, how badly *do* you want to be well? Jesus often asked questions when people came to Him for answers, so I thought I would use the same method here with you. Jesus knew what Legion's name was, but He asked anyway. He knew how long the epileptic boy had been afflicted, but He asked the father anyway. He asked the disciples who people said that He was, but He already knew the answer. Jesus also knew that the blind man wanted his sight restored, and yet He asked him, "What do you want Me to do for you?"

I believe I already know why you are holding this book in your hands. You want to walk in wellness, or if you are already well, you want to stay that way. But by my asking how badly you want it, you get to hear yourself answer the question. To help you out, I will pose it in a different way:

> *Are you willing to do whatever it takes to walk in health with your Healer so that you can be well for as long as you live?*

You see, you have a responsibility in wellness. And wellness merely means "the state of being in good health, especially as an actively pursued goal."[1] So, if you are going to walk in wellness, then that means you are actively going to pursue the goal of being in good health. It means you have a relationship with your own health, as well as with your Healer. You are either going to pay attention to your health, your Healer and His instructions for health and healing, or you are not. It is your choice, and I cannot make it for you. But it is my experience that if people really want to do something, they will do it. If they do not, they will not.

I am not talking about you being perfect, but about you merely making a promise. Not an ungodly promise that leads to stress if you fail, but a holy vow to yourself and to God so that you can proceed with sobriety and succeed. If you can hear yourself say right here, right now that you are going to do whatever it takes to live out all your days here on earth and not let anything or anyone steal even one day from you, I believe you will do it.

God did not have you invest your money, time and energy into this book just to have you back out, give up or shut down before you are done. Nor did He have me write this book so you could read it and forget everything in it. I care for you, friend, but my time is too valuable, my lessons too costly and my wisdom too hard-earned for it all to be so easily tossed aside. The same could be said of you. Your time, lessons and hard-earned wisdom are all waiting and ready for you to put them to work here.

God had me write this book so that you could *know* He wills you well. And so that you can become dissatisfied with being out of His will for wellness and discover His instructions

1. *English Oxford Living Dictionaries*, s.v. "Wellness," accessed July 16, 2018, https://en.oxforddictionaries.com/definition/wellness.

for divine health. I do not know where you are in your descent toward disease or how severe your situation is. You may be reading this book and consider yourself generally healthy, but you just want to make more changes that will take you into vibrant health. Or you may be in a desperate situation and in need of a miracle. Either way, my goal is the same. I want to help you get well . . . soon.

You may be someone who receives a miracle as you read this book, but then what? If God saves you from sin and forgives you, do you then return to that sin? I certainly hope not! Likewise, when you receive a bodily or emotional miracle while reading these pages, you will never again return to the practices that may have contributed to your sickness to begin with. Jesus does want to heal you, but He also wants you to walk in divine health. There is a difference. The latter requires you to cooperate with God and allow Him lordship of your diet. The payoffs are big, though, providing you with much more than just a miracle in one part of your body. Rather, the result is total temple health for a lifetime. After all, your body is the *temple* of the Holy Spirit: "Or do you not know that your body is a temple of the Holy Spirit within you, whom you have from God? You are not your own, for you were bought with a price. So glorify God in your body" (1 Corinthians 6:19–20).

Yes, Jesus loves healing people supernaturally. In fact, He has healed me supernaturally so many times that I have many stories to tell you about it in the pages to come. He does not want you repeatedly at death's door your whole life, having to put everyone who knows you through the time and resource-eating agony of almost losing a loved one. Notice I did not say *ever*, because we all know He can often be glorified through those eleventh-hour miracles. But He is not trying to subject you to a constant barrage of new afflictions that define your life. So as He frees you from certain medical conditions while you are making your way through this book—whether naturally

21

or supernaturally—you must not be like the fool who returns to his folly, if your situation was brought about by things you did or did not do. Or like the dog that returns to its vomit, or the sow that, after washing herself, returns to wallow in the mire (see 2 Peter 2:22). You are not a fool, a dog or a pig. You are a child of God.

Let me put it this way: God *wants* you as His child. He wants to be your Father and to have a closer walk with you. You may have bought this book or may have gotten it as a gift and do not realize yet that you were born to be a child of God. Maybe your mother is His child, or your grandmother is, but you say you are not. I have good news for you. God has no grandchildren. Just children. He created you for a purpose that no one else on earth can fulfill, and if you do not stay alive and healthy enough to fulfill it, the earth or someone on it will feel the void. This world is full of such felt voids. It is full of people too sick to fulfill their purposes. For every individual not fulfilling a divine purpose, there is someone else out there in danger of missing his or hers because of it. You must stay well. You must have a relationship with your health and with your Healer. Knowing good nutrition keeps you out of trouble. Knowing the Healer gets you out of trouble when it comes. But wouldn't you rather it never come?

It is with tears in my eyes and sobriety in my heart that I begin this book. It is almost as if I can hear the conversations of desperate, sick people in my ears. It started today, as I merely disembarked from a plane and headed toward the baggage claim. I have been contracted to write this book for many weeks now and have been in constant prayer and planning. Just today, however, the tangible mantle came to begin the work, and it fell on me in the middle of a busy, bustling airport. While leaving the plane and entering the gate, I suddenly felt this indescribable compassion wash over me as I began hearing what must have been a global cry for healing. I literally heard one person after the other, for one reason or another, lifting their petitions up to the Father for help. People on their knees or in healing lines, by their hospital beds or on bathroom floors in their homes. I saw one mother with beautiful dark, curly hair praying for her child to be healed. The prayers swelled so loudly that I could no longer make out the words. But I knew all these people were praying the same prayer at different times and in different languages: *Please heal, God.*

I began to cry as I literally heard these cries for help. I am certain people saw me and thought I was distraught. The truth is, I was. Distraught for you. Do you, or does someone you love, need healing in body? I hear you. Do you need greater energy and less fatigue? I hear you. Do you need hormonal balance and your youthful vigor back? I hear you. Do you need a stronger back and neck, with pain-free rest? I hear you. Do you need to get to sleep more quickly each night and stay asleep? I hear you. Do you have internal organs that are in need of creative, reconstructive miracles, or maybe joints that ache more often than not? I can hear you out there. Do you have emotional struggles that have left you anxious, depressed and even suicidal? I hear you. Have you had a diagnosis that is trying to define your life, ruin it or even end it? I hear you, I hear you, I hear you. I am here to help you. Jesus is here to help you. The three of us will make a great team to get you back on your feet again. Jesus and I are going to do all we can to get you healthy, but we need your help. That is why I began this book by asking you how badly you wanted vibrant health.

And now I am going to make *you* a promise . . . a simple vow. I know that Matthew 5 tells us not to swear falsely or take unnecessary oaths and to just let our yes be yes and our no be no. But vows are a very godly concept, and you need to hear me make this one to you. I have not written this book to give you false hope. This is not a book that overpromises and underdelivers. You and I both know people who pursued healing and health and never got it. It is part of living in a fallen world that has never regained its footing after plummeting from the perfection of total body, mind and spirit health. But here is why I am expectant for you: *Heaven has inspired me to write a book that not only opens the door for your healing, but that also closes off every door to illness.* We are going to call down miracles and then help you learn to maintain them. I *know* this book is different than any other book out there, (1) because of the comprehensive body, mind and spirit approach to healing and staying healthy, and (2) because we are going to both bless all your body systems and teach you to feed them as a means of prevention against further illness.

I can also hear those of you out there who are currently healthy. You are saying that you want to do whatever it takes to stay healthy in this disease-riddled world. Or perhaps you are committed to an industry or a ministry that helps others find health and healing. Either way, good for you!

I have to say this, and I bet you will agree: I am so weary of people around me dying of sickness. Or even just struggling with sickness. I hate sickness. I detest it with everything I am, and I have devoted my life to helping others live out the fullness of their days the way God intends. The thing I am most looking forward to in heaven—after seeing Jesus, my grandparents, the prophet Elijah, author Ellen G. White (whom I call the nineteenth-century health prophetess) and my dear friend Pastor Sheila—is that we will all be living in a place where *everyone* is healthy. Totally whole. I have interviewed and listened to people who died, went to heaven and then came back, and they tell me that they had an awareness of having a body there. So imagine it: Each one there will be (and is already) standing tall, with a healthy back, breathing freely, glowing with healthy skin and bright eyes, fully energized, with a healthy heart, and with no internal or external maladies. Nor any emotional nor spiritual wounds. Imagine living in such a place. It is God's will!

And now consider this: In the Lord's prayer, we pray for God's will to be done "on earth as it is in heaven" (Matthew 6:10), right? Well then, I want to try to help people walk in that divine health *here*. I believe it is a worthy aim that would not detract one bit from heaven's experience and reality. In fact, I believe when more people see Christians walking in divine health, they will want to become Christians. And then think how much more full heaven could be. Yes, your good health is a witness to others.

In the meantime, so is your recovery process. Most of the world is recovering from something, so never let the enemy tell you that you cannot be an effective witness for God while waiting. Why would Scripture tell us to practice patience if we never had to wait on anything? And why would there be a need for the 1 Corinthians 12 gifts of working of miracles and gifts of healing if there were never any sick people or desperate needs for miracles? God is glorified through *all things* . . . in both the absence *and* presence of sickness.

I just want a stronger army for God as soon as possible. Don't you? We need evangelists who can travel free from the restraints of pain and infirmity, apostles who can live to be quite old so they can share all their wisdom with the churches they plant, pastors who are not so sick and out of shape or overweight that they are too tired to tend God's flock at a moment's notice, teachers who can burn the midnight oil when necessary in order to receive priceless revelation from God before teaching, and prophets who are so healed emotionally that they prophesy God's words, not their own words coming through a filter clogged from past wounds and rejections. And now imagine each one of these people raising up others just like himself or herself to join the ranks. Now *that* is an army that is able to concentrate on God's Word and be led entirely by His Spirit, without limitation!

By the time you finish this book, each of your 15 body systems will be thoroughly blessed, and any sicknesses you have will be prayed over. Yet in order for this to have any amount of lasting fruit, you must look at the body system blessings and healing prayers in part two as seeds, and therefore give ample attention to the soil, weeds and climate of your life before and after planting them. Here is how we will accomplish that:

1. Here in part one, I will introduce you to ten steps (one step per chapter in these first ten chapters) that will ensure the proper planting, watering and weeding of the seed blessings and prayers in part two.

2. Then in part two, you will remind yourself of these ten steps via a declaration you will make before receiving each body system blessing. It will be important for you to hear yourself reiterating these steps, or for others whom you are praying the blessing over to hear themselves declaring them.

3. After each body system blessing, but before the healing prayer for that system, I will introduce you to an "A-list" of advice that will help you maintain your miracle, or will get you the rest of the way there. The A-list includes foods to *avoid*, foods to *add*, supplements to *allow*, essential oils to *apply*, a directive to daily *anoint* yourself, and a reminder to *ask* your health care provider before making any changes to your regimen. Be smart with this advice, but do not let it replace the counsel of your personal doctor, nutritionist or health care provider. Rather, incorporate it with their blessing, explaining to them that you are pursuing vibrant health in body, mind and spirit.

It is that simple. And how do you find the body system blessing or healing prayer you need? One of two ways: (1) If you are relatively healthy and are looking to prevent sickness, then you will find your way to the body system you want blessed through the table of contents at the front of the book. (2) If you are in need of healing, you will look up the sickness that has already attacked your body system by searching the alphabetized illness index at the back of the book. The index will connect you with your healing prayer. I guess you could say that the healthy will come in through the front door, and the sick will come in through the back door. But both will wind up at the same place.

I see this book being kept at church altars so when the sick come for prayer, ministers and intercessors can just pray the appropriate healing prayer and read the appropriate body system blessing over the person in need. Both the prayer and the blessing will contain great physiological detail about how that part of a person's body should be functioning—not so we can impress God with our medical terminology, but so both the giver and the recipient will feel great authority rise up as they pray in agreement for the body to function as God once created it to do.

So often when prayers for healing are being prayed, either the giver or the recipient is secretly doubting what the will of God is for that situation. He or she holds back or never fully believes for healing, which is the surest recipe for not receiving anything, according to Jesus' own words in Mark 11:24: "Therefore I tell you, whatever you ask in prayer, believe that you have received it, and it will be yours." We must *believe*, or why pray at all? But we also must know and understand God's will in order to be able to believe. As Ephesians 5:17 says, "Therefore do not be foolish, but understand what the will of the Lord is." With part two's body system blessings and healing prayers, there will be no question as to what the will of God is for the body of the person being prayed for. He created everything to function in an ordained way, which each recipient will discover in great medical detail during the prayer. Also, every symptom of the illness will be addressed and dismissed. Great faith will arise as a result of this understanding and agreement.

Citations and references are crucial to any book with medical information. I cited as many as fifty sources in my previous books, but this project feels different. For instance, the body system blessings and healing prayers in part two are chock-full of medical terminology and research, yet for me to litter the prayers with endless footnotes would have been very distracting to you whenever you are trying to pray those prayers and listen to the Holy Spirit (especially if you or the person you are praying with is in pain). So I have decided just to disclose my main sources up front. Doing that will ensure a more user-friendly flow throughout the rest of the book, which is imperative in a prayer setting, especially if you are sick and in no frame of mind to be flipping to endnotes. Here is my three-pronged approach to this project's citations:

1. I relied heavily on Mayo Clinic, mayoclinic.org, as I have for many years. I remain impressed with Mayo Clinic for multiple reasons. Not just because of the expansive staff of physicians, scientists and other medical experts, and not just because of the website's impressive lineup of medical editors, which ensures great accountability. But because every disease has its own staff and medical editor, and in some cases (such as with cancer) multiple medical editors. Plus, all the clinic's doctors and medical experts dedicate a portion of their clinical time to mayoclinic.org, so that means the public is getting direct access to the knowledge, research and experience of Mayo Clinic. Also, every medical editor is either an M.D., R.N., Ph.D. or a combination of those, sporting more letters *after* his or her name than *in* it. That is also the case, by the way, with Dr. Jim Sharps, N.D., H.D., Dr.N.Sc., Ph.D., the president and CEO of

the International Institute of Original Medicine (IIOM, my alma mater) and the writer of this book's foreword. He would never endorse a book that did not have a truthful body, mind and spirit message, so his backing of this project speaks volumes.

2. I also relied on WebMD, webmd.com, and WebMD's sister site, onhealth.com. The experts involved have created one of the most comprehensive learning environments for all things medical on the Internet today, providing credible information, support communities and in-depth reference material about health issues you need to know about. The website says, "The WebMD content staff blends award-winning expertise in journalism, content creation, community services, expert commentary, and medical review to give our users a variety of ways to find what they are looking for."[2] You could get lost on WebMD for hours, and I sometimes do. And yes, those experts come with plenty of letters after their names, too.

3. Finally, speaking of letters after your name, I have some new ones after mine, in case you missed them on the cover. I now have my master's degree in Original Medicine, and I am in graduate school again for my doctorate in Original Medicine. When I am done, I will be an N.D., a naturopathic doctor. I have no current plans or desire to hang out a shingle and open a practice. In fact, the only reason I am furthering my education is for *you*. I want to be able to help you by providing you with all the resources you need to make better decisions for your body, mind and spirit. That is what Original

2. "About WebMD: What We Do for Our Users," WebMD, last updated April 29, 2014, https://www.webmd.com/about-webmd-policies/about-what-we-do -for-our-users.

Medicine is—God's design for body, mind and spirit health—and His is the only path to wholeness. I believe that if I can at least set you on that path—and cheerlead you along the way—you will make the right decisions. And always remember that it is your doctor or health care professional who knows the story of your whole body. I do not. Always ask him or her before you make changes to your medical regimen. Together, we all make a great team to get you healthy.

Once again, friend, I have heard you. Have you heard me? Then we are ready to get to work! In whatever way and from wherever you arrive at a particular body system in chapters 11 to 26, you are in for a blessing. A total temple makeover. Or maybe you are not laden with multiple maladies and you just want better overall health. Either way, this book is for you. Are you ready? Tell God just how ready you are. Then we will move on to chapter 2, where you will take inventory of your health.

2

Take Inventory of Your Health

Body, Mind and Spirit

I f this is the first Laura Harris Smith book you have ever read, you may not be familiar with how I define health. I do not believe that you can claim to be healthy at all unless you are nurturing your body, your mind and your spirit, but to do that, you have to first be aware that you even have a body, a mind and a spirit. You have to be awakened to the reality that you are a triune miracle. And for those of us who *are* awakened to it, it is amazing how quickly we can forget it in our day-to-day activities.

Take for example what you are doing right now. Look at your hands that are holding this book or device as you read it (and don't worry about that manicure you need or the age spots you despise). Consider that without your eyes, you would be unable to see those hands (or hangnails and age spots), or ingest what you are reading. If you are listening to the audiobook, consider that you are doing so because you have ears that are doing their jobs. But once you ingest the information you are reading or listening to, where does it go? It goes into your mind. You read and process, read and process, and before you know it, you have learned something new. Your body will benefit from what your mind retained. And most people stop there.

But very few people let their spirit read a book. *And how do you do that?* you ask. You will need to know how before you can accurately take inventory of your body, mind and spirit health and be blessed in your entire being through the enclosed prayers, so we will try a simple exercise. The Holy Spirit is waiting right now for you to give Him access to that eternal part of you that is longing for His touch.

Okay, stop. Did you catch that? You just read that last sentence the way you always do—with your mind—but now I want you to read it again with your spirit, paying special attention to the permissions you are giving, or not giving, the Holy Spirit as you read:

The Holy Spirit is waiting right now for you to give Him access to that eternal part of you that is longing for His touch.

Now close your eyes for a few seconds and picture that a literal Person is sitting beside you—the Person of the Holy Spirit. Go ahead. I will be waiting right here whenever you reopen your eyes. . . .

Okay, the last part of that italicized sentence said He is waiting for you to give Him access to an eternal part of you. And not only that, but it says that it is the part of you that is longing for His touch. Did you even know that you are longing for something? Are you in tune with what your spirit man or woman needs? Are you even aware that there is an eternal part of you that is currently walking around incarcerated in your temporal body? That body will only live so long, right? But your spirit will live forever. And you get to choose now if your spirit will live with God once you die, or live entirely separated from

Him in eternal darkness. He will never impose Himself on you, whether in life, in death or even when reading this book. But whatever and wherever you choose, you *are* going to live forever, and forever is a long time. Therefore, forever requires investment. Forever requires you to give it access. Forever begins right now. So invest in forever by reading this book with your spirit.

How do you do that? You will feel the Holy Spirit near you if you will pause occasionally and give Him permission to speak as certain statements nudge you. This book is—and all my books are—intentionally full of such unspoken opportunities for pauses and permissions. They are not marked out for you, but if you will be mindful of the Holy Spirit's nudging as you read and take time to pause anywhere that stands out to you, He will know He has permission to work further in that area. If you will do that, you will get the most out of each blessing spoken over you and each prayer you pray for yourself.

Now then, if this is *not* your first Laura Harris Smith book, you already have a keen understanding of the body, mind and spirit axis that defines you. You know that this trifold axis and how you care for it dictates the outcome of your health, both good and bad. You believe in the Trinity, a triune being comprised of the Father, Son and Holy Spirit, and you know that He is not 1+1+1=3, but 1x1x1=1.

Furthermore, you believe that this unfathomable miracle is alive in you *right now* because you are made in His image. It is more rare than the phenomenon of identical triplets—a comparison I often make that still falls short, but is the best a human can do! You will recognize this from Genesis 1:26, in the Garden of Eden, when the triune nature of God is first revealed as He is making man and says, "Let Us make man in Our image, according to Our likeness" (NASB). You know that the "Us" and "Our" the Father is referring to is none other than the Son and the Holy Spirit, and that, of course, the same Trinity miracle is also represented in His beautiful masterpiece called *woman*, because Genesis 1:27 says, "God created man in His own image, in the image of God He created him; male and female He created *them*" (NASB, emphasis added). You also know that this threefold miracle is replicated each time man and woman unite together and create new life, and that this replication has happened without exception for all the billions of people who have ever been born on this earth throughout its history.

If you have read my prior books, you know this is what I firmly believe and have thereby intentionally built my body, mind and spirit ministry upon. Hopefully by now you believe it, too, and have benefited from this ministry and these truths. Whether you are male or female, this supernatural Trinity created you in His image to be a lesser trinity here on earth that serves as His reflection. You cannot reject His DNA inside you any more than you can crawl back into your mother's womb and refuse conception.

Now that you and I are sure we are on the same page about how to define health—body, mind and spirit—we can take inventory of *your health*. Here is how we will accomplish that: In the following list of physical, emotional and spiritual needs, place a checkmark in each box that you feel describes a statement you would make about yourself. (Remember, you can download this same checklist free at lauraharrissmith.com/forms, if you would rather write on that instead of in the book.) In the margin to the left of each box you check, list the month and year you recall that your symptoms began. (This will be important and helpful information in a later chapter.) Once you go through this checklist, you will know exactly how to navigate through the prayers and declarations in part two as they are offered to you.

Physical Needs

___ I need a healing in my central nervous system (brain, spinal cord, nerves, etc.).

___ I need a healing in my sensory system (sight, hearing, feeling, smelling, tasting, balance, etc.).

___ I need a healing in my endocrine system (hypothalamus, pituitary, thyroid, adrenals, pineal body, etc.).

___ I need a healing in my circulatory system (blood, all vessels, etc.).

___ I need a healing in my cardiovascular system (heart, blood vessels: arteries, capillaries, veins, etc.).

___ I need a healing in my respiratory system (lungs, nose, pharynx, larynx, trachea, bronchi, alveoli, etc.).

___ I need a healing in my digestive system (mouth, esophagus, stomach, liver, gallbladder, small intestines, etc.).

___ I need a healing in my excretory system (large intestines, colon, rectum, etc.).

___ I need a healing in my urinary system (kidneys, bladder, etc.).

___ I need a healing in my reproductive system (ovaries, testes, uterus, etc.).

___ I need a healing in my skeletal system (bones, joints, teeth, cartilage, etc.).

___ I need a healing in my muscular system (muscles, ligaments, tendons, etc.).

___ I need a healing in my immune system (bone marrow, thymus, glands)

___ I need a healing in my lymphatic system (spleen, lymph nodes, ducts, tonsils, etc.).

___ I need a healing in my integumentary system (skin, hair, nails, sweat glands, etc.).

___ I need healing from a sleep disorder (insomnia, sleep apnea, narcolepsy, etc.).

___ I need healing from a genetic or congenital disorder.

__ I need healing from a metabolic disorder.

__ I need healing from a chemical mental imbalance.

__ I need healing from an autoimmune disease.

__ I need healing from weight gain, obesity, anorexia or bulimia.

__ I need healing from allergies.

__ I need healing from chronic infections.

__ I need healing from unexplained infertility.

__ I need healing from being crippled or lame.

Emotional Needs

✓ I need better emotional health overall.

✓ I need healing from depression.

✓ I need healing from grief.

✓ I need healing from anxiety.

__ I need healing from anger or rage.

__ I need healing from paranoia or schizophrenia.

✓ I need healing from fear or worry.

__ I need healing from jealousy.

__ I need healing from hate.

__ I need healing from prejudices.

✓ I need healing from guilt and regret.

✓ I need healing from distrust.

✓ I need healing from shame.

✓ I need healing from disappointment.

✓ I need healing from constant discouragement.

✓ I need healing from hopelessness and despair.

✓ I need healing from previous memories.

__ I need healing from pride.

✓ I need healing from loneliness.

✓ I need healing from disorganization and lack of focus.

___ I need healing from discontentment.

___ I need healing from greed.

___ I need healing from being imprudent and unwise.

___ I need healing from control and domination.

___ I need healing from inferiority and insecurity.

___ I need healing from self-loathing.

Spiritual Needs

___ I need healing from anger at God.

___ I need healing from feeling unloved or forgotten by God.

✓ I need healing from distrusting clergy and church leaders.

___ I need healing from the spirit of unforgiveness.

___ I need deliverance from the spirit of doubt/unbelief.

___ I need deliverance from being easily offended.

___ I need deliverance from the spirit of rebellion.

___ I need deliverance from substance abuse or addiction.

___ I need deliverance from lust or a pornography addiction.

___ I need deliverance from the spirit of mental illness.

___ I need deliverance from the spirit of idolatry.

___ I need deliverance from nightmares or night torments.

___ I need deliverance from the spirit of suicide or murder.

___ I need deliverance from the spirit of witchcraft.

___ I need deliverance from the spirit of sexual perversion.

___ I need deliverance from the spirit of poverty.

___ I need deliverance from the spirit of isolation.

___ I need deliverance from the spirit of failure.

___ I need deliverance from the spirit of death.

___ I need deliverance from the spirit of hypocrisy.

___ I need deliverance from a lying spirit.

___ I need deliverance from the spirit of gluttony.

___ I need deliverance from the spirit of materialism.

___ I need deliverance from the spirit of workaholism.

___ I need deliverance from unidentified demonic influences.

___ I need deliverance from various torments.

You may need to refer back to this checklist as you pray through this book. In chapter 1 you expressed to God your readiness for vibrant health. In this chapter, you have taken inventory of your health in its current state. The next step, just ahead in chapter 3, is going to require your cooperation and honesty.

3

Acknowledge That God Did Not Make You Sick

Of utmost importance in moving toward vibrant health is acknowledging that anything short of it is not God's fault. We see that disease is not God's idea, because there was no such thing created for Adam and Eve in the Garden of Eden. Upon finishing creation, God said *it is good*, and part of that goodness was a disease-free world. No sicknesses were present through which He could conspire intentionally to discipline, punish or mature humankind through suffering into His perfect image (a common misconception). Maturation is definitely a by-product of suffering, but God does not sit and plot about how He might visit hardships on the immature. His design for free will prohibits such manipulation.

No, God wanted a well world. Imperfect infirmity only invaded perfect creation once sin invaded. But we will discuss that more in the next chapter, as you learn more about taking personal responsibility for your health. For now, it is vital that you are convinced that health is God's best for all of humankind, including you. Health and healing are sometimes hard enough to attain without thinking God is against the idea.

Not only is any current lack of health in your body, mind or spirit not God's fault; it is also not His best for your future. One false teaching that has a deadly stronghold on the Church says that God sometimes strikes His children with sicknesses to teach them lessons or to see how much more strongly they can learn to depend on Him. I cannot imagine any good earthly father who would adopt such abusive behavior, much less a perfect heavenly Father. Matthew 7:11 says, "If you then, who are evil, know how to give good gifts to your children, how much more will your Father who is in heaven give good things to those who ask him!"

Still, I was one who believed this false doctrine, and I spent many years in chronic sickness, believing there was no hope for me. I take full responsibility since I was well versed in Scripture and could have, at any time, seen that God offers healing in both the Old and New Covenants. He actually introduces Himself to us in Scripture as Jehovah Rapha, which literally means in Hebrew "*the God who heals*" (see Exodus 15:26). His very name shows that healing is not just something He does; it is who He *is*. Psalm 103:3 tells you that God "heals all your diseases."

Jesus carries on His Father's healing ministry. We see in Matthew 4:23 that He went about "healing every disease and every affliction among the people." We also know that we are to carry on this same ministry, because we are told in Matthew 10:8, "Heal the sick . . ." And James 5:14–15 tells us that if any among us are sick, that person is to call for the elders of the church to anoint him (or her) with oil, and that the prayer offered in faith will make the sick person well. These few verses are just appetizers for you in an entire Bible menu of healing Scriptures and stories for you to feast upon.

Unfortunately, many have pointed out one opposing passage in particular on which to hang their unbelieving hats for an argument against God's desire to heal all His children. I know, because

I once used it to explain why my healing from violent convulsions had not come. It is Paul's thorn passage in 2 Corinthians 12. In my book *The 30-Day Faith Detox: Renew Your Mind, Cleanse Your Body, Heal Your Spirit* (Chosen, 2016), I spend three of the thirty daily devotionals dissecting this controversial passage in an attempt to forever lay to rest the gross misinterpretation of Paul's words in the original Greek, which has caused so many Christians to settle into their sickness as if it were God's idea. I am sure I was not the first to offer corrected teaching on this passage, but since I had not heard it taught anywhere, I felt the obligation to address it. I would like to recap it quickly here in just a moment, but I invite you to get *The 30-Day Faith Detox* and study the teaching in full on Days 15, 16 and 17 for yourself, if for no other reason than to kick down fully this abominable doctrine that ruins God's good name and breaks His Father's heart.

But what about God allowing certain illnesses, even though He did not directly cause them? you ask. As I always say to suffering Christians who ask that, God was not on vacation when this happened to you, so it obviously passed through His hand and He allowed it. But if you will let Scripture interpret Scripture in the original languages, and not rely on your own interpretations of a few passages here or there, your faith will find new footing for healing and your circumstances will change.

Friend, if you have asked God for healing and it does not immediately come, you are faced with two choices. You can (1) believe that God has given you a life sentence (or worse, a trip to death row) and ask for extra grace to muddle through it. Or you can (2) accept His biblical invitation to engage in spiritual warfare, surround yourself with an army of saints who will fight with you, employ some basic laws of nutritional health, and then ask for extra grace to stand your ground. My life and health did not change for the better until I did the latter.

But what about those who do all those things and don't recover? you may ask. In chapter 27, "Troubleshooting Stubborn

Illnesses," we will definitely explore the reasons why healing sometimes does not come. But first, I want to do that recap of my three-day teaching on the controversial Paul's thorn passage. If you have been among those who believed that if healing does not come after you have asked God three times for it (or fewer), it must be His will for you to remain sick, then that wrong mindset ends today for you. I ask you merely to look at what God's Word says in the original Greek, and then open your heart to some good news. *The* Good News.

> So to keep me from becoming conceited because of the surpassing greatness of the revelations, a *thorn* was *given* me in the *flesh*, a *messenger* of Satan to harass me, to keep me from becoming conceited. Three times I pleaded with the Lord about this, that it should leave me. But he said to me, "My grace is sufficient for you, for my power is made perfect in weakness." Therefore I will boast all the more gladly of my *weaknesses*, so that the power of Christ may rest upon me.
>
> 2 Corinthians 12:7–9, emphasis added

Countless Christians—after reading flawed commentaries or hearing inaccurate teachings by favorite, well-meaning pastors—have interpreted it like this:

> So in order to keep me from being conceited, God gave me a disease, inspired by Satan, to torment me. Three times I begged God to take the disease from me and He refused, telling me grace was enough and that He wanted me to stay sick. Therefore, I will brag about being sick and weak for Jesus.
>
> 2 Corinthians 12:7–9, MCT
> (the Misled Christian's Translation!)

You may be among those who think my MCT version is farfetched, but it is much more likely that you are among those who know it is not. Or you may be living under this unnecessary yoke right now, and I wish I could crawl through the pages of this book and hold you! But what you need much more than a hug is to hear God's Word divided correctly, because "faith comes by hearing, and hearing by the word of God" (Romans 10:17 NKJV). Where there is poor teaching on what God's Word actually says, there is little faith in it, and Matthew tells us, "Anything is possible for someone who has faith!" (Mark 9:23 CEV). What is the opposite of "anything"? *Nothing.* So reverse that verse and you have "Nothing is possible for someone who has no faith." On the topic of healing, we *must* activate your faith, and to do that, according to Romans 10:17, we must let you hear the Word of God, and you must hear it accurately.

Refer back to the 2 Corinthians 12:7–9 passage and let's take a look at the words I italicized for you there, because by defining them in the original Greek language Paul penned them in and putting them back together, we can learn exactly what this important passage is teaching us. Although Paul was not imprisoned when he wrote these words, many have tried to imprison the words themselves, probably in an attempt to explain why some people are not healed. How sad, because as a result, they have imprisoned the Good News itself. Pay close attention to these definitions[1] of the italicized words from 2 Corinthians 12:7–9:

> *Thorn:* Greek *skolops*, meaning "a stake" or "a thorn." Only used once in Scripture. Paul's thorn was metaphorical and not literal, or he would have used *akantha*, the word for Jesus' crown of "thorns."

> *Given:* Greek *didōmi*, meaning "to give, to give over, to intrust." Also used in Matthew 16:19: "And I will give [*didōmi*] unto thee the keys of the kingdom of heaven: and whatsoever thou shalt

---

1. All Greek word definitions here are taken from the Blue Letter Bible's lexicon at https://www.blueletterbible.org.

bind on earth shall be bound in heaven: and whatsoever thou shalt loose on earth shall be loosed in heaven" (KJV). And in Luke 10:19: "Behold, I give [*didōmi*] unto you power to tread on serpents and scorpions, and over all the power of the enemy: and nothing shall by any means hurt you" (KJV).

Flesh: Greek *sarx*, meaning everything from "the soft substance of the living body, which covers the bones and is permeated with blood of both man and beasts" to "mere human nature, the earthly nature of man apart from divine influence, and therefore prone to sin and opposed to God."

Messenger: Greek *aggelos*, meaning "a messenger, envoy, one who is sent, an angel, a messenger from God." Appears 186 times in the New Testament. In 179 of these citations, it is translated "angel." In 7 times, it is translated "messenger." It is never a thing, disease or object. It is always a living being.

Weakness: Greek *astheneia*, meaning "of the soul; want of strength and capacity; to bear trials and troubles," or "want of strength, weakness, infirmity; of the body, its native weakness and frailty, feebleness of health or sickness." Some translations use the word *illness* in place of *weakness*, and yet nowhere is that found in the original Greek.

From these definitions we can draw the following conclusions:

1. *God is the giver of the "thorn in the flesh," not Satan.* While this seems to contradict my earlier defense of God as the loving Father, not to mention offend my fellow full-gospel friends, understanding that God is the giver of the thorn is a vital part of this passage. In the opening words of verse 7, Paul reveals the giver's motive: "to keep me from becoming conceited." So I ask you, do you really think Satan wanted to keep Paul's pride in check? Would

the devil like to keep Paul from sinning? No. God must be the giver of this thorn. Paul's heavenly revelations were so grand that God gave him the thorn to keep him humble, and it accomplished just that. Paul was certainly full of humility. If we let Scripture interpret Scripture, however, we will come to verse 7 with this already established truth from Matthew 7:11 in mind: "If you then, who are evil, know how to give good gifts to your children, how much more will your Father who is in heaven give good things to those who ask him!" From this and many similar passages, we know that if God gives a thorn, we must explore exactly what it is, since it *cannot* be a bad gift that will result in bad things. It would be unscriptural, ungodly and unfatherly, according to God's own words about Himself, and God *never* contradicts His Word. So then, what was Paul's thorn? That leads us to #2.

2. The *"thorn in the flesh, a messenger of Satan to harass me"* is a demonic principality or spirit, not an illness or infirmity. Each of the 186 appearances of the word *aggelos* in Scripture always describes a living, feeling being— never an object or a thing. Paul's thorn in the flesh was not a "what" at all (including a sickness), but a "who." Remember that the fullness of that word's definition also includes "messenger, one who is sent, an angel." Since the actual Bible text reads "a messenger [*aggelos*] of Satan," we see clearly that this must have been a dark angel, "a messenger of Satan sent to harass." In fact, the Weymouth New Testament translation of 2 Corinthians 12:8 says, "As for this, three times have I besought the Lord to rid me of *him*" (emphasis added). Not "rid me of *it*." The thorn was a *him*! Paul was begging God to deliver him from the constant interaction with this demonic opponent. Why would God not do that for Paul? And why would a good

Father "give" a messenger of Satan to Paul at all? The exciting answer is found in #3.

3. *God "intrusted" and "gave over" this demonic being to Paul in order for him to take authority over it and subdue it in the earth.* We just defined that the Greek word in the phrase "was given me" is *didōmi,* which, among other things, means "to give over, to intrust." This demon was sent by God and "given over" to Paul. It was entrusted (modern spelling) to him. But for what? For Paul to defeat it, to have authority over it and to grow in his understanding of his authority over other such dark messengers. Paul was a thorn in *his* side. This entity had no authority over Paul, for God would never allow a demon to be in authority over one of His children. Remember Job? God did not allow Satan to test him to keep him from sinning, but to prove to Satan that Job would *not* sin (and he did not). Same with Paul. I am convinced that in the end, God's plan was for Paul to learn that this demon—and others like him—were under his authority. How else does God take dominion over spirits of darkness on the earth, if not through His children? We are what He has to work with down here! In fact, this *didōmi* word is the same exact *give* word used in these other Bible passages about God giving Christians authority over evil spirits: "Behold, I give [*didōmi*] unto you power to tread on serpents and scorpions, and over all the power of the enemy: and nothing shall by any means hurt you" (Luke 10:19 KJV). "And I will give [*didōmi*] unto thee the keys of the kingdom of heaven: and whatsoever thou shalt bind on earth shall be bound in heaven: and whatsoever thou shalt loose on earth shall be loosed in heaven" (Matthew 16:19 KJV). If you still believe that Paul's thorn/messenger was a sickness, you surely will not think so after reading #4.

4. *Paul did not have a chronic illness; the "flesh" that Paul says his thorn-messenger was in was not his physical body.* Remember that *sarx* (Greek for *flesh*) is a body *or* mind word. Its meaning carries both body and mind characteristics (see the previous definitions again). Those who believe this thorn was a bodily disease claim *sarx* as only a body word, and most of those argue that Paul had an eyesight defect. They point for this to some biblical evidence of Paul's impaired vision through the "large letters" of his handwriting, the Galatians' willingness to have plucked out their own eyes and given them to Paul, and his failure to recognize the high priest (see Galatians 6:11; 4:15; Acts 23:1–5). Their theory is that Paul asked God three times to rid him of this chronic eye ailment and that God refused him, stating that His grace was sufficient for him to remain visually impaired. But others—myself included—believe Paul also intended *sarx* as a mind word here, referring to the part of the Greek definition that says "human nature, the early nature of man apart from divine influence." So when he said *skolops sarx* (translated "thorn in my flesh"), he was using a metaphorical term to describe an inner struggle that yes, may or may not have had physical manifestations. But if you are among those who still think Paul had a chronic vision infirmity based on that Galatians 4:15 passage, where he references the Galatian people being willing to pluck out their eyes for him, I offer you another perspective. If you follow the timeline of Paul's journeys at the time of his writings, it is easy to see that in Galatians 4, Paul is discussing the stoning in Lystra (in Turkey), which he endured in Acts 14:19–20, just before coming to Galatia. The stoning was so brutal that Paul was presumed dead, but then verse 20 says that as the disciples stood around him, he somehow arose, and he left the next day with Barnabas

for Galatia (Derbe). Both ancient and modern scholars agree that the Galatian churches were in south Galatia, and that any traveler coming from Lystra (Turkey) would have had to pass through the Cilician Gates (in Turkey) and wind up in Galatia. Thus, my theory is that Paul arrived in Galatia weak in body and mind after this horrific Lystra stoning, and that this was the *astheneia*, the weakness, he referred to in Galatians 4:13. He would have journeyed the sixty miles from Lystra to Galatia in this badly injured condition, a journey that would have taken three days over rough terrain, which was at best an unpaved track. He was badly in need of recovery, and who knows, maybe he even needed a new set of eyes if his assailants had aimed at his face (which was common). This would explain Paul saying that the Galatians were willing to give him their eyes. You may say, *Well, if Paul was stoned so badly then, why doesn't he ever mention wounds or scarring on this same journey?* My answer is . . . he did! Just two chapters later, he says, "For I bear on my body the scars that show I belong to Jesus" (Galatians 6:17 NLT). So do you see that this was *not* an ongoing, chronic illness? For people to believe that the Galatians 4:13 passage insinuates a chronic infirmity, they must first be predisposed to the wrong thinking that Paul was chronically ill. Unfortunately, the folks who think that way point to 2 Corinthian's thorn passage, stating that he was continuously sick because of God thrice refusing him healing. But notice again the previously mentioned Galatians 4:13, where Paul says his infirmity was "at the first," indicating that it was not a permanent ailment at all, but something temporary that he had arrived with (like wounds from a stoning), which mended and healed during his stay. He was weak "at the first," but then recovered. Case closed.

5. *Paul's thorn* (skolop) *and his infirmities* (astheneia) *were the dangers and persecutions he suffered because of the Gospel.* He said in 2 Corinthians 12:9 (NKJV) that he would boast in his "infirmities"—plural—so if you are going to claim that Paul had one chronic disease, you are going to have to claim that he had several, because of how often this word is used in Scripture. Examples of these uses of *astheneias* are in Acts 9:23, 26–29; 13:6–12, 44–50; 14:1–19; 16:12–40; 17:1–14; 18:1–23; 19:23–31; 20:3. I highly suggest that you take five minutes to look them all up. Further proof that this thorn in the flesh was not a chronic illness is that all the scholars who emphatically claim this is a physical illness cannot even agree on what it was. Epilepsy? Malaria? Leprosy? Depression? Headaches? Stuttering? Hysteria? Ophthalmic eye disease? For heaven's sake! The reason they cannot agree on an illness is because it was not an illness at all. Paul was not ill; he was under demonic attack by a spiritual antagonist. For those who still insist that these "infirmities" were chronic sicknesses, it should be noted that almost every major translation of the Bible chose the word *weaknesses* and not *infirmities* in translating, including the NIV, NASB, ESV, NLT, HCSB, ISV, NET, ASV, GW, ERV, DARBY translation and more. Pure and simple, Paul's persecutions made him weak at times. Do you ever feel weak during persecution against you? Of course you do. It bears repeating that *weakness* is the Greek *astheneia* and means "want of strength, weakness, infirmity; of the body, its native weakness and frailty, feebleness of health or sickness." The word also means "of the soul; want of strength and capacity; to bear trials and troubles." Combined, these meanings suggest someone who is *weak in body and mind because of trials and trouble.* The overall meaning points directly to that gruesome stoning Paul

49

had just received. True, the Greek definition offers the options of "sickness," but I imagine that Paul's stonings, fastings and nakedness in the cold did make him sick (not to mention "seasick"), don't you? This is further proven in 2 Corinthians 11, where he details his infirmities (*astheneias*), none of which are chronic illnesses:

> Three times I was beaten with rods, once I was pelted with stones, three times I was shipwrecked, I spent a night and a day in the open sea, I have been constantly on the move. I have been in danger from rivers, in danger from bandits, in danger from my fellow Jews, in danger from Gentiles; in danger in the city, in danger in the country, in danger at sea; and in danger from false believers. I have labored and toiled and have often gone without sleep; I have known hunger and thirst and have often gone without food; I have been cold and naked. Besides everything else, I face daily the pressure of my concern for all the churches. Who is weak [*astheneō*—root of *astheneias*], and I do not feel weak [*astheneō*]? . . . If I must boast, I will boast of the things that show my weakness [*astheneias*].
>
> 2 Corinthians 11:25–30 NIV

Did you catch that in the last two verses? Paul refers to all these trials as astheneias, and you can clearly see that these persecutions and dangers were not chronic illnesses. Since this is the same exact word he chose in the famous 2 Corinthians 12:9 (NKJV) thorn passage, "I will rather boast in my infirmities [astheneias]," we can know that Paul was not saying he would boast in a chronic sickness (as some do today, wearing their sickness like a badge), but in the chronic persecutions and dangers he overcame one by one. He even echoes this again in the 2 Corinthians 11 passage you just read, where he says, "If I must boast, I will boast of the things that show my weakness [astheneias]" (verse 30). Again, there are a very few translations that choose the word infirmities here and say "I will boast in my infirmities," but note that 21 of the major Bible translations use the words weakness or weak. Mystery solved!

6. *God did not deliver Paul from the demonic harassment when he asked, because God does not deliver us from persecution.* Jesus told us that persecution would come to us, as it came to Him. We cannot rebuke it. And Paul echoes this in 2 Timothy 3:12: "Yea, and all that will live godly in Christ Jesus shall suffer persecution" (KJV). But God's grace is sufficient for us, just as it was sufficient for Jesus and Paul. And consider this: If God ended all persecution, Saul would never have become Paul. Stephen was stoned to death, and Acts 7:58 says of the encounter, "Then they dragged him out of the city and began to stone him; and the witnesses laid their coats at the feet of a young man named Saul" (NRSV). In chapter 8 Saul is still persecuting Christians, but at the start of chapter 9 he has his Damascus Road encounter and is reborn into Paul. But it all began with Stephen's persecution and stoning. I hope you see from this study of the original Greek language that the thorn in Paul's flesh was persecution. Persecution from a messenger of darkness who influenced many ungodly men to torture Paul. They tried to prevent Paul from preaching the Gospel, yet it made him cling to it all the more. In fact, they even imprisoned him, yet each incarceration only provided him more time to pen another epistle for us. God's grace was indeed sufficient for Paul, just as He assured him it was in 2 Corinthians 12:8.

Remember that the expressions "thorn in my flesh" or "thorn in my side" did not originate with Paul. In the Old

Testament, this phrase referenced an aggravation with the ungodly. In Numbers 33:55 Moses says, "But if ye will not drive out the inhabitants of the land from before you; then it shall come to pass, that those which ye let remain of them shall be *pricks in your eyes, and thorns in your sides*, and shall vex you in the land wherein ye dwell" (KJV, emphasis added). Joshua 23:13 says, "They shall be snares and traps unto you, and *scourges in your sides*, and *thorns in your eyes*" (KJV, emphasis added). And Judges 2:3 says, "They shall be as *thorns in your sides*, and their gods shall be a snare unto you" (KJV, emphasis added).

Did Moses, Joshua or Samuel literally have thorns in their sides or their eyes? No, and neither did Paul. Did Moses, Joshua or Samuel mean that they were physically ill? No, and neither did Paul. He was the Pharisee of Pharisees. He would have known about this scriptural phraseology and would have drawn from it. He used this phrase because he knew God had told Moses that if he would not drive out these ungodly inhabitants, they would become a vexation to Israel.

Likewise, if you do not drive out the ungodly inhabitants in your life—those demonic forces that are trying to make you sick, keep you sick *or tempt you to make poor health choices*—you will also have thorns in your flesh. You have authority over them. God entrusts to you the power to overcome the world. He also gives you the power to overcome your own bad choices that could affect your health. Now that we have determined that you truly want to be healthy, and we have taken inventory of your health and acknowledged that God did not make you sick, we can move forward into our next chapter, which will help you attempt to discover the root of your condition.

4

Discover the Root
of Your Condition

For you to move toward vibrant health, you must discover how you moved away from it. Unless your ailment is congenital (from birth) or an injury (leaving you disabled), it very well could be that your choices have landed you where you are. In our previous chapter, we discussed how God did not make you sick and how it is not His best for you to stay sick. That begs the question, *Then who or what does make me sick?*

We just read how sometimes a spiritual force of evil can result in an attack on our wellness and well-being. But more often than not, it is not the enemy, but our own bad choices that affect our health.

Simply put, sometimes we have no other choice than to look in the mirror and take personal *responsibility* for our poor health. I want you to look closely at that word *responsibility*.

Response-Ability

How will you *respond* to the *ability* God has given you to make changes? As you make your way through this book, you will have responses to everything you read. Responses are internal, good or bad. For example, you might decide, *I like that strategy.* Or you might think, *That statement offends me.* But what you do with those *responses* will demonstrate your *ability* to bring about change in your life. So govern your responses carefully and wisely. Tell them who is boss. Remember what you learned in chapter 1 about reading this book with your spirit? That will make managing your responses easier. Then you will discover greater ability to act on those responses and make real change occur in your body and mind.

If the component of reading something with your spirit has been missing in your past, it would be why you may have read many books, articles or even helpful nutritional emails and texts from friends, but they wound up not working for you. You responded with excitement and hope at first, but there seemed to be no follow-through. There was a breakdown somewhere between your *response* and your *ability*. Thus, you never took real *responsibility*.

What good would it do a person in a medical emergency to have a team of first responders show up early but have no ability? Or what good would it be to have the best first responder team show up . . . late? You have to have both response and ability. I have worded the sentences, paragraphs and chapters of this book in such a way as to provoke responses from you. Then I give you plenty of ideas to increase your ability to follow through. So let's put that to the test right now. What is your response when I say the following? *Sickness and sin are related.*

In chapter 3 we discussed how God created a world without sickness, and how disease only invaded our world once the door was opened to it through sin. There is no escaping the fact that sin and sickness are related. It is not a popular statement, and it is especially uncompassionate if someone says it to the suffering. Nonetheless, it is an inconvenient truth. More than once when Jesus healed or rescued a person, He said, "Go and sin no more." What an odd, even rude thing to say to a sick person, or even a newly restored person. But Jesus understood the sin/sickness relationship. He understood that it is actually uncompassionate *not to educate* people to the connection between their soul and body.

Can you imagine how you would feel if, after being dramatically healed by the touch of Jesus Himself along His path in Galilee, and standing there with grateful tears in your eyes, He turned to you and said, "Okay now, enough with the sinning." Or, "Hey, no more of that thing that got you here to begin with. Got it?" Man, oh man. I think I would rather have Jesus spit in my eyes with mud, as He did with the blind guy in Scripture. Or maybe I would rather be Lazarus, who was left dead in the tomb for four days. But no way would I want Jesus reminding me of my sin at a moment like that. And especially not in front of everybody else.

And what about today? Can you imagine how offended you would be if your doctor gave you a clean bill of health after your recovery and then added, "But don't sin and mess this up!" I would be so offended that I would probably find a new doctor, but not before writing and deleting a long, career-stopping Facebook post that would never see the light of day. But Jesus did not mind offending people for their own good. He even went so far as to say to the lame man in John 5, "See, you are well! Sin no more, so that nothing worse may happen to you" (verse 14). Jesus also said something similar to the woman caught in adultery. He had no problem warning people of the dangers of sin. One of these people was lame, and the other was being stoned. Their choices had landed them in need of the Healer because the wages of sin is death (see Romans 6:23).

So why are we surprised today when our life choices land us in need of the Healer? It stands to reason that we should get to know Him and walk in health before sickness ever comes. Psalm 103:2–3 says, "Bless the LORD, O my soul, and forget not all his benefits, who forgives all your iniquity, who heals all your diseases," which also lends biblical credence to the fact that there is a sin/sickness relationship.

Granted, this is not to say that everyone who is sick is in that situation because of personal sin. Sometimes it is generational sin or the fact that we live in a fallen world where sin seeks to invade and erode everything, including the health of the innocent. We will explore this more in chapter 6, "Unleash the Blessing (and Reverse the Curse)," and also in chapter 27, "Troubleshooting Stubborn Illnesses."

The bottom line, however, is that disease manifests in one of three places: your body, your mind or your spirit. But it always originates in the spirit. Here is why I say that: You are a triune being made in the image of the Trinity, so to be whole, you must have a revelation of the connection between all three of these components that make *you* you. Where the spirit is healthy, there will be a relationship with God in which you hear His voice, so you will have better emotional health (in the form of joy and purpose). But you will also experience better physical health because that same voice of guidance will help you make healthier choices for your body and help you feel the spirit of conviction when you do not, which prompts change.

When a person's spirit is unhealthy, it often goes unnoticed until a symptom manifests in the mind (anxiety, depression, etc.) or in the body (through disease). When I say *mind*, by the way, this category includes "the mind, will and emotions," as does the Greek word from which *mind* originates, *psyche*. Dr. Caroline Leaf and others teach that the brain includes both physiological issues (such as mental illnesses and chemical imbalances) and emotional ones (such as depression). Many people treat their physical or emotional symptoms and never stop to seek God's spiritual counsel on the root of the matter. They are treating only one-third or two-thirds of themselves and will never be whole. Good physical and emotional health begins with a healthy spirit.

So then, you might ask, *Why do Christians ever get sick?* The answer is very simple. Just because you are a Christian does not mean you are spiritually healthy. Just because Jesus is your Savior does not mean He is your Lord. That is a totally separate surrender, and just because you have asked Him for eternal life does not mean that you allow Him to govern your earthly life. He has your heart, but not your fork. These poor health choices do not cost you your eternal life. In fact, it is just the opposite. You will get to heaven sooner!

Conversely, just because you look healthy on the outside does not mean you are healthy on the inside. Poor spiritual health will eventually catch up with you by manifesting in another realm. For example, you hear of people all the time who run five miles a day, then drop dead of a heart attack. My opinion? This seemingly healthy runner may have been running from something emotional that put an intense, hidden strain on his or her heart, relationships and attitude toward God. The runner's "heart disease" was of a spiritual nature and eventually manifested in his body. He looked healthy and fit on the outside, but was rotting away on the inside.

Or practically speaking, perhaps this person was not running from anything at all emotionally, and his or her heart attack had a very physical explanation. He had paid great attention to his cardiovascular health and to staying fit, but had ignored wisdom on how unsafe it is to eat large amounts of meat before running, because the strain on the body to digest that food during such physical exertion could result in death.

Either way, a healthy spirit would have prevented the heart attack. How? In the first case, a healthy spirit would have brought emotional peace to this runner and resulted in lower stress and better cardiovascular health. And in the latter case, a healthy spirit would have given him access to the voice and wisdom of God, and as he made the poor food choices before running, the Spirit of God would have warned him. A healthy spirit always precedes a healthy body and mind.

For decades, science has been suggesting that disease is rooted in our emotions, heartaches, bitterness and disappointments. I call it "emotion sickness," and just like motion sickness, you cannot go very far down the road until you slow down and address what is causing your lack of ease (dis-ease). Negative emotions are said to contribute to death, not to mention premature aging and chronic illness. For example, it is thought that envy is linked to arthritis. I believe Scripture backs this up in Proverbs 14:30: "A tranquil heart gives life to the flesh, but envy makes the bones rot."

Dr. Chris D. Meletis is highly respected internationally as an educator, physician, author and lecturer. At the age of thirty, he became the chief medical officer and dean of clinical education at the oldest naturopathic medical school in the United States and was given the 2003 Physician of the Year Award by the American Association of Naturopathic Physicians. His personal motto is "Changing the world's health one person at a time," and he believes that when individuals become educated about their mind and body, that is the moment when true change begins. He addresses this concept of emotion sickness on his website in the article "It is True that 'Stress Kills.'" In the article, he says that over and over again in his seventeen-year clinical practice he has seen that ignoring your feelings can literally destroy you from the inside out and erode away your health.[1] He references a case study done by the *Journal of Psychosomatic Research*:

---

1. Chris D. Meletis, "It is True that 'Stress Kills,'" iHeathScience, 2017, https://www.ihealthcast.com/?p=93.

Extreme suppression of anger was the most commonly identified characteristic of 160 breast cancer patients who were given
a detailed psychological interview and self-administered ques-
tionnaire. Repressing anger magnified exposure to physiological
stress, thereby increasing the risk of cancer.[2]

And then he quotes the international journal *Cancer Nursing*:

Extremely low anger scores have been noted in numerous
studies of patients with cancer. Such low scores suggest suppression, repression, or restraint of anger. There is evidence
to show that suppressed anger can be a precursor to the development of cancer and also a factor in its progression after
diagnosis.[3]

That is the effect of *suppressed* anger, but *outbursts* of anger
are evidently a precursor to heart attacks. In the 2015 CBS
News report "Angry outburst could trigger heart attack within
hours," Dr. Thomas Buckley, a senior lecturer and researcher
from the University of Sydney and Royal North Shore Hospital
in Australia, says that the increased risk of heart attack after
intense anger or anxiety is "most likely the result of increased
heart rate and blood pressure, tightening of blood vessels
and increased clotting, all associated with triggering of heart
attacks."[4] I believe that Ecclesiastes 7:9 (NRSV) confirms this:
"Do not be quick to anger, for anger lodges in the bosom of
fools." I would say that the heart is in the "bosom," wouldn't
you? Do not let anger lodge in your bosom.

Here are the steps I want you to take to discover the root of
your condition. Return to your health inventory checklist from

2. Ibid.
3. Ibid.
4. Robert Preidt, "Angry outburst could trigger heart attack within hours,"
CBS News, February 24, 2015, https://www.cbsnews.com/news/angry-outbursts
-could-trigger-heart-attacks/.

chapter 2. In the left margin you wrote the month and year of the onset of your condition's symptoms, to the best of your memory. Now your investigative work begins: (You can grab a piece of paper to jot down your revelations as you proceed, or you can download and print this in work-sheet form for your convenience at lauraharrissmith.com/forms.)

1. Get somewhere quiet and ask the Holy Spirit to remind you of the events going on in your life during or prior to when you first noticed your symptoms (difficult or painful events occurring as much as one year prior).

2. To boost your memory, check previous calendars—both electronic and old paper calendars (if the symptoms began that long ago)—to remind yourself of your involvements at that time. List those.

3. If calendars are unavailable, scroll through old email inboxes and sent mail to spark your memory of life events taking place during that time. List those.

4. If your symptoms and condition began long before you kept calendars or had email, interview friends or family members, or look through old diaries, pictures or journals for clues. Even old report cards or changes in school grades for the worse might form a picture of what happened for you.

5. Ask the Holy Spirit to bring to mind the dates or seasons of any difficult relationships or heart wounds, without dredging up anger or unnecessary pain. We are merely trying to find any true correlations between your emotional struggles and your physical conditions. Depending on the severity of the symptoms and condition, they could take up to a year to manifest physically after an emotional or spiritual trauma, so really investigate your timeline to get to the root.

6. If you get any clues from the above steps, draw a timeline on a piece of paper that connects these emotions and illnesses in a linear fashion, so you can see your life laid out before you in a straight line. (You can also print out a timeline that I designed for you at lauraharris smith.com/forms. This is separate from the work sheet you printed out earlier for this exercise and will prove a helpful addition.)

7. If you remember an emotional trauma or a serious life event that could have had a negative emotional impact, yet no physical condition manifested during that time, go ahead and write that emotion or life event on top of the timeline without linking it to anything else.

8. Now your healing work can begin. Look for connections along your timeline of difficult life events and sicknesses.

9. Starting with the events on the top of your timeline, make a forgiveness list with names of people you need to forgive and release to the Holy Spirit. (A forgiveness list form is also available at lauraharrissmith.com/forms.)

10. Make another list of people who need to forgive *you*; people whom you may have sinned against or who *think you did* in the midst of these traumatic life events or seasons. Even if you did not sin against them, just knowing that others think you did so can be a heavy weight on your soul over time. (Download a form for this list, too, at lauraharrissmith.com/forms.)

11. Pray through each name on the list of those people whom you need to forgive, really taking time to forgive those whose actions and decisions had a negative impact on your life.

12. Pray and ask God to forgive *you* for times when you or your decisions had a negative impact on the life of

another. Go to each individual whom you feel needs to hear your apology. Your willingness to do this could have a major impact on the health of those individuals, so do not rule it out.

13. Thank God for the good things that came from that situation or relationship you are thinking of, asking Him to help you remember only the good and release to Him the bad.

14. If it is warmer weather, sit outside and burn your forgiveness lists, then scatter the ashes or bury them at the base of a favorite tree or plant. In cooler weather, do this indoors in a fireplace, garage or well-ventilated, safe area.

In this chapter you have explored the reasons and roots of your condition. As we discussed, sometimes sickness is rooted in spiritual or emotional trauma, and sometimes it is related to sin. Sometimes that sin is not your own, but generational sin that can be cleansed from your family line. (We will discuss that more in chapter 27, "Troubleshooting Stubborn Illnesses.") But always ask God to examine your own heart for areas that are not fully submitted to Him. Even the smallest of transgressions that may have opened a door to the devil can make the enemy think he has a legal right to afflict you. As you can see in #10 in the previous list, there is a transitional point after you have been sinned against at which you can enter into sin yourself. It is at the point when you choose not to forgive that the door is opened to strife-induced sickness. Unforgiveness is the predecessor to countless tormenting illnesses and difficulties. Jesus warned us of this in Matthew 18:34–35 (DARBY):

> And his lord being angry delivered him to the tormentors till he paid all that was owing to him. Thus also my heavenly Father

shall do to you if ye forgive not from your hearts every one his brother.

This is absolutely astonishing to me, that our loving heavenly Father is so firm with us about what will happen if we do not forgive. And yet many of us do not. One of the saddest biblical truths has got to be the number of saved, churchgoing, Bible-reading, Sunday school–teaching Christians who are in the hands of tormentors. I know some. Do you? Let's not be one of them. Ask the Father for grace to forgive.

Now that you have decided how well you want to be, have taken inventory of your health, have acknowledged that God did not make you sick and have explored what may be the root of your condition(s), let's move onward to dealing with your doubt. We all have a bit of it crouching at the door, just waiting to sneak in. Let's see how you are doing with it.

5

Pray the Prayer of Faith

The prayer of faith for healing is comprised of four distinct directives. See if you can find them in James 5:14–16:

Is anyone among you sick? Let him call for the elders of the church, and let them pray over him, anointing him with oil in the name of the Lord. And the prayer of faith will save the one who is sick, and the Lord will raise him up. And if he has committed sins, he will be forgiven. Therefore, confess your sins to one another and pray for one another, that you may be healed. The prayer of a righteous person has great power as it is working.

1. *You yourself call for others to come pray.* This is not to say that others cannot initiate praying for you without your asking (or that you cannot initiate praying for someone else), but when a person is sick, there is something faith-activating about the process of asking others to come and pray for you. By the time you have done that, you have decided you are truly ready for change. You have given great thought to those who would be in total spiritual

agreement with you, and you have stepped out in faith toward your future. This decision, forethought, risk and vulnerability all set the stage for expectancy, which is a major component of faith. The praying does not always have to be done by the governmental elders of the church, but just those "elder" in the faith (mature).

2. *Let them pray over you, anointing you with oil.* If you are not familiar with this practice, it is time to become so. All throughout Scripture, anointing oil is used to represent the presence of God, without which the human mind can easily forget the availability of the supernatural when in prayer. Moses anointed Aaron. Samuel anointed Saul and David. Elisha anointed Jehu. Mary anointed Jesus. And there are so many more examples. The disciples "anointed with oil many who were sick and healed them" (Mark 6:13). And disciples are still doing it today. You can anoint on the forehead and on the body part in need of healing (but do be respectful and get permission from the individual first, especially if the person is of the opposite gender). Oil also represents unity, which is needed in a setting where you need to pray in agreement. "Behold, how good and pleasant it is when brothers dwell in unity! It is like the precious oil on the head, running down on the beard, on the beard of Aaron, running down on the collar of his robes!" (Psalm 133:1–2).

3. *Pray in faith.* This means to have faith in God, not faith in your faith. Many get tripped up trying to work up their faith, bringing great distraction to their mind, which should be focusing on God's love for them and His ability to do the impossible. It is less like "great faith" to climb up to, and more like childlike faith to relax into. When this focus is available, the prayer of faith is easy to pray, and the language of your prayer will move from *I believe*

You can to *I believe You will.* For many, it then becomes, *I know You just did; thank You.* The Mark 9:24 prayer is always there for us: *"I believe; help my unbelief!"* Don't rush over or skip this part of the prayer time. It is fine for you to allow ample time in this setting for God to help any unbelief you might be battling, which helps you rediscover the faith of a child as you wait on Him. God is able to handle your doubts, but you must face them and confess them to Him.

4. *Confess and receive forgiveness of sins.* This is not only a good time to confess our doubts in His healing ability, but also our sins in general. Many a person has been healed once confession of sin has taken place. It is as if healing can now fill a geographical spot in the soul that the burden of sin once filled. I myself have experienced dramatic healing after both confession and extending forgiveness to others who had sinned against me—so much that if I am ever experiencing an unusual display of symptoms in my body, I stop and ask myself, *Whom have I not forgiven? What sin have I allowed to creep in?* To be even more transparent, I will confess something to you that happened to me just tonight. I have felt very poorly the last 72 hours. I developed what felt like an abscessed tooth, with a lot of pain (and I have never even had a cavity, so I was a big baby about it). I also injured my back moving furniture by myself and could hardly move without excruciating pain. And I was having horrible stomach pains due to some dietary changes I had made (healthy ones that were evidently causing a healing crisis as my body began purging some toxins). I have been in a mental fog for three days. Then tonight, I heard from someone by email about how I had greatly offended her recently (the email came in while I was writing this chapter). It broke my heart and I had to apologize, confessing

that if I ever got in trouble, it would always be with my mouth! I was able to see this person's point, even though I did not have a clue that I had hurt her. I apologized sincerely tonight because I saw now that I had. I repented and begged forgiveness. I have not even heard back from her just yet (it has only been two hours), but in that short amount of time, my toothache and swelling have entirely gone away, my back has entirely quit hurting (I am touching my toes, jumping, twisting), and my intestinal pain is entirely gone. How can that all be a coincidence? Sin and sickness are linked, friend. I had sinned against a friend, and even though I did not know it, my body somehow knew it, and it manifested with sickness. Transgressions silently knock us off-kilter. Only through the powerful, often missed secret ingredient to this James 5 passage (the confession of sins for healing) did my healing come. This proves that cleansing the soul goes hand in hand with healing the body. In light of this, look at every confrontation from an accuser as a gift—an opportunity for you to look inside your soul and find what may be impeding your healing. So often, people will not come to you when you have wronged them, and of course, Proverbs 19:11 does tell us it is to a man's glory to overlook an offense, so they may be keeping silent in order to obtain a greater measure of God's glory. But what a gift when someone affords you the chance of confession and restoration. It is not that the Lord will withhold healing from you if others do not tell you when you wrong them, and it is not as if you must live a perfect life to be healed, but when a door opens for you to humble yourself and repent, be sure to walk through it. Your healing may be just on the other side.

As I mentioned in chapter 3, I used to suffer from horrible convulsions. Although I was attending a Baptist church at which

I never remember hearing a teaching on physical healing, I knew these leaders loved me and would do anything to see me in better health. So I asked my dear pastor about this James 5 passage. We did not have "elders," but I asked him whom we could have gather to pray for me, and he told me he would be happy to ask the deacons. My husband, Chris, and I scheduled a time later that week to meet with a few deacons and the pastor in his office. I can still remember when he pulled out that bottle of anointing oil. I was 25 years old and had never seen one. As far as I knew, an angel had hand-delivered it to the pastor that afternoon. The fear of the Lord washed over me. Sounds silly now, but when you do not even know that anointing oil exists (much less is sold to the public), you feel as though you are in the middle of a holy moment just by looking at it. I was glad I had come. That meeting changed my life.

But it did not change my health. What happened? I cannot speak for everyone else in the room, but I can for myself. Although I had done #1 (called for others to pray over me) and although they had done #2 (prayed and anointed me with oil), I honestly do not think #3 or #4 occurred. I think I prayed the prayer of hope, but not the prayer of faith. I did not know God's Word as I do now about how He longs to heal His children, so our prayers that night sounded more like *Lord, if it be Your will*, instead of *Lord, I see in Your Word that healing is Your will*. I also never engaged in any kind of confession of sin. I cannot remember the details or condition of my soul at that time (my mind, will and emotions), and I do know that I was daily striving to please the Lord, but that matters not. We all sin. We all hold grudges. We all covet. We all speak loosely sometimes. We all sin and fall short of the glory of God (see Romans 3:23). God must know this if He names confession as an element necessary for healing: "Therefore, confess your sins to one another and pray for one another, that you may be healed" (James 5:16).

The meeting did not necessarily feel rushed, but James 5 is very clear that the way for healing to transpire in that setting is for the prayer of faith to be prayed and for the confession of sins to occur. If it takes a long while to understand and accomplish those, then a long while must be allotted. Surely it does not compare to the time spent being ill, missing work, researching cures and suffering.

At Eastgate Creative Christian Fellowship, the church we planted and pastor in Nashville, we have time at the end of every service for anyone to come and receive prayer for healing. Miracles are not uncommon, large and small. We have what we call an "A-Team," an altar team comprised of elders, deacons and other intercessors. They come forward and line the altar as Chris closes the service every Sunday. People come and ask for prayer, and by doing so, they have accomplished #1. While there, they are anointed with oil, which is #2. You can bet that the prayer of faith is prayed, #3. And when our leaders' gifts of healing are met with the recipient's gift of faith (see 1 Corinthians 12), amazing things happen. In this beautiful setting, the confession of sin almost comes naturally. People experience God's presence and cannot help themselves. It is beautiful. I cannot count the people who have come forward for a healing miracle, and while receiving prayer have wound up confessing how their poor eating habits got them into this mess. I also cannot count the times that someone comes forward for one thing and winds up confessing another. An affair. A drug addiction. A grudge. Big or small, step #4 is a vital part of the equation and cannot be overlooked. When coupled with the prayer of faith, look out!

But like you, we have both given and received prayer where healing was delayed or did not come at all. As promised, we will discuss such delays in chapter 27. But there is more work to be done to prepare you for how you will process each of the body system blessings coming your way in part two. First things first. I will tell you for sure that the Lord is near to those who are waiting on Him and trusting Him with the timing of their healing. Just this morning, my devotional was on John 20:29: "Jesus said to him, 'Have you believed because you have seen me? Blessed are those who have not seen and yet have believed.'"

I do not think it was any coincidence that the Lord put this verse before me today. I think it was for you. He wants you to know that you are literally blessed (or in line for a big blessing) if you have not seen and yet have kept believing. Anybody can believe when they see. But only a few can believe all the more even when they do not see. If that is you, God has not forgotten you. In fact, you have caught His attention all the more. He is working on something big for you. Fear not. Be patient. He has promised you healing and will accomplish it. It will take on varied forms, but it will come. Remember, He is Jehovah Rapha.

Remember the four steps of this chapter as you pray each of the prayers for healing in part two. Suggest (humbly) to your pastor that you even keep a copy of *Get Well Soon* at your church altar or wherever the sick are being prayed for. The very specific and medically detailed prayers will get both the prayer givers and the recipients on the same page, with great results. You can also take this book with you to private sessions where you are asking for prayer from others, especially so you can follow the four steps established for us in the James 5 passage and outlined in this chapter.

You have decided just how well you want to be, have taken inventory of your health, have acknowledged that God did not make you sick, have discovered the root of your condition and have learned how to pray the prayer of faith. Now it is time to learn how to unleash the blessing in your body, mind and spirit.

6

Unleash the Blessing
(and Reverse the Curse)

A blessing is a positive, hope-filled and life-giving statement based on biblical principles and promises, which is spoken over a person, place or thing. Notice I did not say "spoken over a deserving person," for the Bible tells us we must also bless those who curse us. But the blessing is a living, breathing life force that eagerly awaits the command of the giver for it to be unleashed. Until then, it remains captive and useless, but when spoken, it can instantly change a person's day, mood, circumstances or even life.

Does the blessing really live and walk about? Does it really breathe? No, not with legs and lungs, but yes, by the Spirit it can and does. Consider this from Acts 17: "He himself gives life and breath to everything, and he satisfies every need. . . . For in him we live and move and exist. As some of your own poets have said, 'We are his offspring'" (verses 25, 28 NLT). So, I submit to you—also poetically—that the blessing is very much alive in the spirit realm and is awaiting your command. You cannot buy it with money or sell it for profit, but according to Scripture, it *can* be stolen from you, so guard it.

To me, one of the saddest chapters of the Bible is Genesis 27. In it, a scheming mother, Rebekah, decides that she wants her favorite son, Jacob, to receive the blessing of his dying father, Isaac, instead of the firstborn twin brother, Esau, receiving it. It is a story of premeditated deceit and bold-faced lies. Rebekah tells Jacob, the indoorsy son, to go gather some clothes from Esau, the outdoorsy son. That way, he would smell like Esau when he approached their father. Her trickery even went so far as putting hairy goat skin on Jacob's hands and neck, since Esau was a hairy man and Isaac would surely touch his son as he was blessing him.

Rebekah then told Jacob to gather some goats so she could prepare Isaac's favorite meal, to distract him (because you know that the enemy often uses food and appetite to arrange our downfalls). Jacob insisted that he could not do this, lest he be cursed. But his mother said in verse 13 (NLT), "Then let the curse fall on me, my son! Just do what I tell you. Go out and get the goats for me!" What is most interesting about that statement is that a curse did fall on Rebekah. She never saw her favorite son again. Once their scheme was carried out, she had to send Jacob away immediately afterward so he could avoid Esau's wrath.

Verse 38 (NLT) emotionally engages you to the point that you almost feel as if you are in the tent with Esau and his father after Isaac blessed the younger son: "Esau pleaded, 'But do you have only one blessing? Oh my father, bless me, too!' Then Esau broke down and wept." But it mattered not. The firstborn blessing does not get a second chance.

Esau mourned because he knew the importance of the blessing. But wait, did he? Just two chapters earlier, he had returned from working in the fields and found Jacob making red stew. Claiming starvation, he had agreed to sell his birthright for that stew, thereby joining the ranks of many other biblical characters whose appetites for food led to a great sin—Eve, the Israelites and even his father, Isaac, who would soon follow his appetite in the tent with Jacob's goat chops. Also, the name Esau means "red," indicating that not only was he ruddy (from being outside all the time), but that he also obviously loved that red lentil stew.

So, was Esau's blessing stolen or surrendered? Does the fault lie with the deceiver or with the one who was easily deceived? What a mess, and of course just one chapter earlier, in chapter 26, their father had deceived Abimelech and lied about Rebekah being his sister. (Sound familiar? Grandfather Abraham had done the same thing to Abimelech with Sarah in Genesis 20). What a lamentable family legacy. There was obviously a generational curse of lying and deceit that ran through their bloodline. And it cost them dearly.

Yet we never see Isaac rescind Jacob's blessing. The reason is because the blessing cannot be rescinded. Once it is unleashed, it goes to work and brings prosperity and peace. Even if the giver changes his mind, the blessing seems to have a mind of its own once it receives its commission. Even God seemed to honor this truth, because Jacob becomes Israel and transforms into a man of great wealth and influence, not to mention having twelve sons, through one of whom would come the Messiah, the Lion of the Tribe of Judah.

I have told this next story in a previous book, but it is worth retelling. In 2007 I was a part of a prayer team that served at TheCall, a multidenominational, international gathering for Christians everywhere to come to Nashville and worship together. Chris and I had been invited to go to one of the tents set up to receive people for prayer. The tents were themed, and ours was called The Father's Blessing. I remember being a bit disappointed, because I had wanted to be in the Healing Prayer tent since I was sure that was where the miracles would take place. But to my surprise, the line for The Father's Blessing wrapped around the tent and all the way down the hill. It was the longest line at any of the tents. People need the Father blessing, whether it be from their heavenly Father or earthly father. They will stand in line in ninety-degree July sun for it. And there were multigenerational miracles in that tent for sure that day. I will never forget them.

In general, there are plenty of Bible passages that give basic blessings for you to release over others. When in need of one, you can usually turn to chapter 1 of any of Paul's letters. He is attributed with Romans, 1 and 2 Corinthians, Galatians, Ephesians, Philippians, Colossians, 1 and 2 Thessalonians, 1 and 2 Timothy, Titus, Philemon and Hebrews. Go to chapter 1 in any of them and you will find a wonderful blessing hiding inside, because remember, each was a letter to friends and co-laborers in Christ. These believers needed a blessing, and their spiritual father, Paul, was always ready to give it. For example,

> I always thank my God for you because of his grace given you in Christ Jesus. For in him you have been enriched in every way—with all kinds of speech and with all knowledge—God thus confirming our testimony about Christ among you. Therefore you do not lack any spiritual gift as you eagerly wait for our Lord Jesus Christ to be revealed. He will also keep you firm to the end, so that you will be blameless on the day of our Lord Jesus Christ.
>
> 1 Corinthians 1:4–8 NIV

> With this in mind, we constantly pray for you, that our God may make you worthy of his calling, and that by his power he may bring to fruition your every desire for goodness and your every deed prompted by faith. We pray this so that the name of our Lord Jesus may be glorified in you, and you in him, according to the grace of our God and the Lord Jesus Christ.
>
> 2 Thessalonians 1:11–12 NIV

But of course, there were many other biblical blessings that did not originate with Paul, such as 3 John 2 (NIV): "Dear friend, I pray that you may enjoy good health and that all may go well with you, even as your soul is getting along well." And of course, we cannot forget the Aaronic Blessing found in Numbers 6:24–26 (AMP):

> The LORD bless you, and keep you [protect you, sustain you, and guard you]; the LORD make His face shine upon you [with favor], and be gracious to you [surrounding you with lovingkindness]; the LORD lift up His countenance (face) upon you [with divine approval], and give you peace [a tranquil heart and life].

The part two blessings that will be spoken over your entire body, mind and spirit are to be revered and cherished. They were not written lightly and are being spoken over you as if we were there together. So remember the power that is being unleashed as you read them, and when possible, read them out loud each time (and then have me read them over you at lauraharrissmith.com/blessings). Some of you may want to read a particular blessing over a certain part of your body daily, until you see change there. And since the blessings were written and released in a spirit of prayer, meet that with agreement by receiving them in a spirit of prayer. That means getting some place quiet, in an unrushed environment, to read the body system blessings. Put on some worship music to help tune your spirit to the activity of the Holy Spirit, your Healer. *This* is how the blessing will bypass resistance and interference and make its way to you more quickly.

Now that we have discussed blessings, let's look at curses. They are real and are constantly looking for a place to alight. Thankfully, Proverbs 26:2 says, "Like a sparrow in its flitting, like a swallow in its flying, a curse that is causeless does not alight." The analogy is that of a bird circling and unsuccessfully trying to find a place to alight. We hope the curse will do the same thing, be unable to alight, when trying to land upon our lives. The Good News Translation says, "Curses cannot hurt you unless you deserve them. They are like birds that fly by and never light." So the question is, *How on earth do you deserve a curse?* Or, *How can we make sure that any curses trying to find us are causeless?* Maybe first we should identify what a curse is.

The *Oxford Living Dictionary* defines *curse* as "a solemn utterance intended to invoke a supernatural power to inflict harm or punishment on someone or something."[1] *Merriam-Webster* says, "a prayer or invocation for harm or injury to come upon one."[2] Very interesting, because just by defining *curse*, it becomes obvious that we have a supernatural adversary. Otherwise, you would have to believe it is God intending to inflict harm, punishment or injury upon us. Do you believe that? Of course not. No, it is our eternal enemy, Satan, who intends harm to come to us. Daily, as if a desperate actor on a stage seeking an audience, he spews forth endless monologues of curses against us, hoping that just one of them will stick. Even Christians are not exempt from this verbal abuse, although we can become very adept at resisting him and the side effects of this constant tug-of-war. It is when our thoughts or words about ourselves and our bodies or situations line up with his curses that the trouble begins. Then, the curse can be "deserved" because you have given it legal right to be there. You have thrown out the welcome mat for it and agreed with your enemy. Let this never be said of you! Take a look at these verses if you need further convincing:

> From the same mouth come blessing and cursing. My brothers, these things ought not to be so.
>
> James 3:10

1. *English Oxford Living Dictionaries*, s.v. "Curse," accessed July 16, 2018, https://en.oxforddictionaries.com/definition/curse.
2. *Merriam-Webster*, s.v "Curse," accessed July 16, 2018, https://www.merriam-webster.com/dictionary/curse.

They bless with their mouths, but inwardly they curse. Selah.

Psalm 62:4

Christ hath redeemed us from the curse of the law, being made a curse for us: for it is written, Cursed is every one that hangeth on a tree.

Galatians 3:13 KJV

And there shall be no more curse: but the throne of God and of the Lamb shall be in it; and his servants shall serve him.

Revelation 22:3 KJV

We see in those last two verses that Christ has redeemed us from the curse because He became the curse, but this obviously does not mean that the curse has left the earth. That does not happen until the very end, according to Revelation 22:3. There will come a day when there will be no more curse, but that day is not today—sorry. You must live your life leaving no door open that gives the enemy's curses legal right to creep through, either by your actions or words, or by those of a family member in your upline who is in authority over you, or who at one time was. These are what we call generational curses, and Exodus 20 (the Ten Commandments) defines them perfectly: "For I the LORD your God am a jealous God, visiting the iniquity of the fathers on the children to the third and the fourth generation of those who hate me" (verse 5).

Surely you understand that as sinful humans we carry a debt toward God. It is the basis and reason for the cross. When we access the cross through salvation, we have propitiation for our sin and can stand debt free before Him. But when the cross is left unaccessed, there is no automatic cleansing for individuals or families. When families have a history of denying God, the curse has a legal right to land there. The proverbial bird from

Proverbs 26:2 does not have to fly far to find a child or grand-child to alight upon, and it is happy to nest in the branches of your family tree.

Or perhaps it is not that a family denies God. Perhaps it is that they welcome both God and sin, in which case a curse still has been given legal right to exist there. It is what we just read in Psalm 62:4: "They bless with their mouths, but inwardly they curse." The blessing and curse will be perpetually at war with one another in families like this—that is, until one family member finally steps forward to be the repairer of the breach through prayer. This individual is someone who gains height-ened discernment and revelation about the generational trouble in his or her family and what it has cost them, coupled with a righteous anger that rises up inside to say, "The buck stops here!" And then this person begins the process of praying over the "sins of the fathers" and educating his or her children, grandchildren, nieces and nephews about the future. The per-son revisits that Exodus 20 passage and claims verse 6: "But I lavish unfailing love for a thousand generations on those who love me and obey my commands" (NLT). He or she begins to place a heavy emphasis on loving God by obeying His com-mands and crying out for His lavish love and blessings.

Such individuals are tide turners in their families. If this is you, you will experience a period of feeling as though you are swimming upstream. Even family gatherings may be hard if you are the only Christian in your family, or if you are the only Christian with a heart bent toward seeing your family receive its full generational blessings. But do not give up! Serve your family. Withstand being misunderstood and forgive them—and yourself when necessary. Just because you have a heart to see your family walking fully in all the blessings God has for them does not mean that you have all the answers. Sometimes all you have is the "want to" and the childlike faith. It is enough. God will do the rest. And much of what you are doing is for your family's downline.

As an example, perhaps a father struggles with pornography. It goes unconfessed and undealt with, and even if he is a Christian, a curse has become deserved and alights upon his family line because of the sin he welcomed. It may not cost him his salvation, but it still robs unfathomable blessings and opens the door to untold thievery. The enemy, well aware of Exodus 20, declares that he is allowed to visit the sins of the father on the children, and so, history repeats itself.

But maybe it is not that this man's son battles pornography, but adultery. It is that same spirit of sexual perversion, but with a different manifestation. And then, if it is still undealt with and unrepented of, with no changes being made, the enemy stands his ground for yet that third generation. Only this time, perhaps it is not pornography or adultery at all that this grandchild embraces, but homosexuality.

Again, it is the same spirit of sexual perversion, just with another hairdo for another generation, which also makes it harder to track and expose. Sadly, if it does land here with homosexuality, although that person can have a loving and sincere relationship with someone he or she considers a same-sex soul mate, the person most likely will be childless. Thus, the original sins of the father—undealt with and unturned from—have now ended his family line. The curse was deserved, it alighted and it severed a family tree.

I have seen this story play out again and again. The enemy comes to rob and kill, but he does not stop there. He also wants to utterly destroy. And he loves destroying families. Why? Because he does not have one. Do not let him join yours.

Next, sometimes the generational curse is not a sin at all, but a family sickness. Perhaps diabetes runs in your family, or cancer. This is why in each blessing we release in part two, we will also reverse the curse of disease that may be in your family.

You will do it in the declaration you make before you receive your body system blessing. Just remind the enemy that God pours out His lavish love to a thousand generations to those who love Him and obey His commands, and then you will take back your family's health.

Now that you have decided just how well you want to be, have taken inventory of your health, have acknowledged that God did not make you sick, have discovered the root of your condition, have learned how to pray the prayer of faith and have prepared yourself for the unleashing of the blessing, it is time to learn the importance of letting your words line up with everything that will be prayed and spoken over you in the chapters to come.

7

Watch Your Words

Lips, be thoughtful, mouth, be wise
Tongue, be fully circumcised
Words, be whittled with a knife
Censor all that is not life

Hand, be ready to move in
Cover death from nose to chin
Mouth, be moistened, smile, don't frown!
Blessings flow where curses drown
© 2001 by Laura Harris Smith

You would never dream of spending hours at the grocery store, filling up several carts' worth of food, only to dump it all out on the floor just before leaving because you did not want to carry the load to the car. And you would never plant a large crop, water and nourish it, then rip up the seed just because it was taking too long to grow. Yet people do these things every day when they destroy with their mouths what they planted and paid for with their faith. I have seen people go to church, receive the instruction of God's Word, pray with great faith and declare with great authority . . . only to curse God in impatience and pitch a fit because He is being too slow. To be honest, who among us has not done that? At least a dozen times?

But I have learned over the years that it does no good. It is a huge setback and just wastes time, not to mention giving the enemy his favorite entertainment: you in distress and angry at God. I sometimes picture Satan and his cohorts sitting around watching my life play out like a movie. Whenever I am tempted to be discouraged or impatient, I make a conscious decision that if I cannot control my circumstances, I can at least control his—meaning that I refuse to be his evening entertainment. Satan's favorite movie is *Curse God and Die*. Mine is *Praise God and Wait*. I am not perfect at it yet, but I am being perfected and have come a long way. In the past I may have even allowed a double feature of both movies on any given day when trial and heartache came. But once you walk long enough with the Father to see Him come through time and time again, it grows easier and easier just to trust Him, praise Him in advance and get busy doing something else in the natural to change your spiraling mood.

Any farmer, including my father, will tell you that crops need more than just seed, water and sun. They need time. And it is the same with every prayer you pray. And it will be the same with every prayer you pray in part two of this book. Some answers will manifest immediately, and others will take time. You cannot just give up because nothing happens and say, "Oh, it is not supposed to be," or "God has forgotten me." No, God is working something out for your good. Be patient with Him and trust that He is hard at work for you. Bigger crops take longer to plant, grow and harvest. Bigger babies take longer to push out. Bigger health struggles sometimes take longer to unravel (some even require multilayered supernatural miracles).

Likewise, bigger prayers that involve multiple individuals require a holy synchronization of parties that only patience can buy you. What you speak during the waiting is vital. Your words must line up with God's. If you instead choose to let them line up with the enemy's, then do not blame God when those careless words come to pass.

For example, sometimes when frustrated, you might be tempted to say, "Of course this would happen to me! It always does!" But look out, because you are sealing your fate when you do that, and you are prophesying more failure and frustration over your future. Your tongue is releasing death, not life, and according to Proverbs, you will now eat its fruit: "Death and life are in the power of the tongue: and they that love it shall eat the fruit thereof" (Proverbs 18:21 KJV). And don't just assume that last part only applies to loving the good fruit. Some people *love* to eat the bad fruit, too. What is eating the bad fruit? Venting. It seems that some people love doing it! Many cannot survive a single day without venting their frustrations out loud. I have done it. You have done it. But if you make a habit of it, you will never prosper. You will live in a constant state of frustration.

When your words do not line up with God's, everything is off-kilter and you will feel it. Like receiving a blood transfusion of the wrong type blood. Or putting regular fuel in a diesel engine. Or giving someone your phone number with one wrong digit. The person will never reach you. And your answer will never reach *you* if you are living this "two steps forward and three steps back" lifestyle. You appear to be doing all the right things and busying yourself to make sure that you do; therefore, it is easy to become indignant with God when you do not get the outcome you worked so hard for. But if you do all the right things while saying all the wrong things (when frustrated or discouraged), you yourself are delaying your answer. You have heard of "walking the walk" and "talking the talk." Well, this is "talking the walk." Never speak death when you are asking God to bring life (and if you want a greater definition of what this means, go read James 1:2–10).

I talk for a living. Whether I am preaching at Eastgate, hosting my television show, *theTHREE* (go to theTHREE.tv to watch archived episodes), or appearing on someone else's show to discuss one of my books, it seems I am always talking. It is not something I choose to do for the limelight or to get attention. In fact, the trait found me when I was very young. My family tells me I was having full conversations on the phone with people when I was eighteen months of age. My parents put me in my first TV commercial at age three, and I would make them endure countless skits that I would write and perform for them at home. The skits always took place in a doorway so I could dart behind a wall, put on a costume and reemerge as a new character.

When my folks started a restaurant, I am told that at age five I would clean the customers' tables before they were done and *ask* for tips, and then I would evidently insert the coins into the jukebox, grab a wooden spoon, stand on another nearby table . . . and sing. I have no recollection of this, by the way, so I will leave it to you to decide if it rings true (which, of course, it does). Once I got in school I always talked too much, and my teachers would check all the related boxes on my report card: "Talks too much." "Needs to listen more attentively." "Talks excessively." But since I always got straight A's, my parents did not seem too worried. In fact, I cannot remember them ever once scolding me about it.

I did try hard to refrain from engaging in so much conversation, but there was so much out there to explore and so many people's stories to discover, and I just had to be at the center of it all. And the real problem was that I could talk and listen at the same time—something that those in charge repeatedly told me was impossible, but I knew I was doing it. So I just tried to learn *when* was the appropriate time to talk. Soon I discovered that the best plan would be just to choose classes that would let me talk, like drama and speech classes. This happened early in life—eighth grade—and I somehow knew I would talk for a living.

What is especially funny is that when I was a TV shopping channel host at Shop at Home TV, I had to wear two devices at all times when on the air. One was a lapel mic for talking, and the other was an earpiece for listening. The producer would talk to me from the sound booth throughout each show, telling me which actions I was doing that were making the phones ring (such as impromptu demonstrations) and then cueing me to return to those actions. This is how big sales happened—by me listening to my producer during the entire show—but the point is that I *had to keep talking while listening.* I remember calling my mother after one of the first shows and saying, "Mama! I am getting paid big bucks to talk and listen at the same time! I told you this gift would come in handy one day! I told you!"

But my point is that when you talk for a living—or talk often, period—you are bound to speak too freely, too unfiltered and too often. Your gift can also be your curse. Or better said, the enemy can try to hijack your gift and turn it into a curse. Simply by the sheer amount of time you spend talking, the odds are greater that you are going to say something wrong, careless or even downright hurtful. I can teach with no notes, preach at a moment's notice and interview people on television without a single question in my head before sitting with them on stage. But I can also speak words that are bombs and not spears, expose someone's wrong motive with no regard for who is overhearing, and be judge, jury and hangman in less than ten seconds flat. In short, I am really skilled at saying the right thing at the right time, but I am equally skilled at saying the right thing at the wrong time—or worse, the wrong thing at the wrong time.

When I was a young mother outnumbered by six children, I learned a lot about myself. Such self-realization inevitably comes with parenthood, but it comes in bucketloads with a half-dozen kids. I was and still am crazy about all my kids. But those six children I was crazy about could literally drive me crazy at a moment's notice! And I did not have the luxury of them being close in age, so that I could occupy them all with the same activity together, put them in bedtime baths at the same time or even discipline them all the same way. No, my six children were spaced over sixteen years, and each day came with the kind of surprises and challenges that result from having to be three places at one time and with a different answer in each one.

For example, I remember one day a potty training mess happened in one room, and in another room was a teenager who had missed a curfew the night before. Downstairs, two of my "middles" were at odds over some inanimate object. Even though my kids were not fighters, hey, if they were living, sleeping, eating and schooling together, then who else's nerves were they going to get on but each other's?

My point is that I could not issue one verdict for all. You cannot ground a toddler or put a teenager in time-out. I remember feeling overwhelmed that day (and many days), but when Laura Harris Smith is overwhelmed, she does not cry and hide in her room with a box of chocolate. Laura Harris Smith gets to the bottom of things quickly and judiciously. I could get things calm and back in order fast, but at the end of some days, I felt as if I had done nothing but issue law and order. So in each room on any given day, I was forced to put on my "think and speak quickly on your feet" hat and issue commands like Judge Judy. But oftentimes by day's end, I would feel as though it was all I had done!

An exaggeration, but outnumbered parents know what I mean. And Chris traveled a lot then, so I often dealt with all of this alone. Thank goodness the kids and I had plenty of snuggles and good talks and closure by bedtime. We saw to it. But God definitely did a lot to refine my gift during that time. I learned that it is not enough to know how to speak articulately. You have to learn how to speak life and not death. And as a mother, I had to learn to be the thermostat in my home and not the thermometer. Anybody can be a thermometer, which measures the atmosphere that is already there and displays it. But to be a thermostat means that you set the bar for what the atmosphere *needs* to be, and you watch the temperature in your home rise to it. It took me years to learn to be a thermostat. It took me years to learn to watch my words with an eagle eye and a discerning heart. My language was not foul, but it often failed those I loved. I felt God's correction each time and always said I was sorry to the one I had failed, trying harder in the next outnumbered moment to speak what should be, instead of what already was. It makes all the difference in the world to your success. And that is experience talking.

Take a look at the following list of "never say" phrases and their alternatives. These are important, whether you are about to vent or even to ask someone for prayer. It is so easy to state the negative. Instead, focus on what God could be doing during the process you are in. (God is big-time into growth.) And remember that His Word is living and active, so memorize ahead of time what you are going to say when trouble comes calling. You will see it flee!

> *Never say:* "I can't get ahead" or "I can't catch a break" or "Nothing ever changes."
>
> *Alternative:* "The enemy is not going to keep me down. I am in God's will, and I will succeed by His grace." (Then make sure you are in God's will.) "I can do all things through him who strengthens me" (Philippians 4:13).

Never say: "Why does this always happen to me?" or "Of course! Bad things always happen to me!"

Alternative: "As of today, this trend in my life ends! I am the head and not the tail, and I am blessed in my coming and going!" (from Deuteronomy 28).

Never say: "God obviously could not care less about my life or my needs. He has forgotten me!"

Alternative: "I just know that God is working this out for me. He has not forgotten me. Isaiah 49:15–16 tells me, 'Can a woman forget her nursing child, and not have compassion on the son of her womb? Surely they may forget, yet I will not forget you. See, I have inscribed you on the palms of My hands'" (NKJV).

Never say: "This person always does this to me. I'm done with this relationship!"

Alternative: "I am going to offer this person the same forgiveness that God offers me. I am going to communicate my needs to him/her and trust God with the outcome. I speak the fruits of the spirit over my life, which include faithfulness, patience and joy" (based on Galatians 5).

Never say: "I can't ever sleep" or "I am an _____ [epileptic, diabetic, cancer, etc.] victim."

Alternative: Speak of these things in the past tense as you fight them. In other words, "In the past I have been unable to sleep, but I know that Psalm 127:2 tells me God gives His beloved sleep. Would you agree with me in prayer about this?" Or "I have been battling seizures [or diabetes or cancer, etc.], but I know God is my Healer. Would you agree with me in prayer for my healing to spring forth speedily?" (from Isaiah 58:8).

You get the point. It is not that you are denying the facts, the sickness or the circumstances surrounding you. You are merely rising above them. You are being the thermostat and not the thermometer. Anyone can say it. You need to pray it. And if you believe these things, then remember to go ahead and thank God in advance. It scares the enemy and reminds him of God's faithfulness, your faith and his inevitable defeat.

At Eastgate, Chris and I hold people accountable to watching their words. It is so easy for friends to vent to each other, but true friends will redirect their conversation toward faith. I always say, "Real friends don't let friends speak death."

Imagine that you had a sword you could wave whenever discouraged. All you had to do was wave it once—whether in the air or at the enemy—and your entire mood and circumstances would change. Well, you do. It is in your mouth. So . . . if you cannot be positive, then at least be quiet. Or read yourself your Miranda rights and tell yourself, *You have the right to remain silent. Anything you say can and will be used against you in a court of law.* Remember, your enemy is listening and watching. Do not become his evening entertainment. This will be *especially* important after you finish the prayers and blessings of part two. Let your words line up with God's Word from the moment you say "amen" to each one.

Now that you have decided just how well you want to be, have taken inventory of your health, have acknowledged that God did not make you sick, have discovered the root of your condition, have learned how to pray the prayer of faith, have prepared yourself for the unleashing of the blessing and have learned to watch your words, it is time in the next chapter to learn what it means to maintain the miracles you are going to get while reading this book.

8

Maintain Your Miracle

While watching your words is one of the main spiritual factors in maintaining your miracle, I want to give you some very practical things you can do in the natural to maintain it. I firmly believe that when you pray the prayers in part two or receive the blessings there, you are going to receive a miracle. If the enemy resists you, you are going to wrestle him for it and enforce the victory that Christ bought for you on the cross. But you must remember not to bring new or continuing disease on your body through poor food choices, improper rest or constant stress.

Let me give you an example. Have you ever heard of someone who eats primarily a plant-based diet with no sugar and no wheat, yet winds up on the brink of diabetes? That was my story. I will briefly recap it here, although you can read the full story in my books *The 30-Day Faith Detox* (Chosen, 2016) and *The Healthy Living Handbook* (Chosen, 2017).

Five years ago, a sleep defiance in which I only allowed myself 4 to 5 hours of sleep a night for years landed me on the brink of adrenal failure. Stage 4 is where all your organs shut down as a result of the loss of the important fuel hormone, adrenaline. By the time I was diagnosed, I was already in stage 3. I was told to make changes or die, and I was put on total bedrest for 3 months. I was also told that if I lived at all, my recovery would take 18–24 months. With some serious lifestyle changes—which included 8 hours of sleep each night and moving to a 75 percent plant-based diet—I fully recovered. And I know there was miraculous intervention, because it happened in only 6 months.

I cut wheat and sugar entirely out of my diet due to how hard they are on the body to process. My organs needed nothing else to do but heal, and they were expending great energy on digesting and absorbing these heavily modified "foods." Not only did my weight drop after cutting them out, but my health also improved quickly. A bonus was that my severe animal allergies and outdoor allergies, which I had suffered with since my teen years, disappeared. Once I totally recovered, I decided to keep sugar and wheat out of my diet. At 53 years old I feel as if I am in my twenties, so why would I want to change that?

Still, unbeknownst to me, I was inheriting another problem I did not foresee. I had replaced wheat flour with mostly rice flour, and I began eating it liberally. Rice crackers, rice bread, rice pasta, on and on. I think I started eating more bread than I ever had as a wheat eater! While my bloodwork had shown just before I cut out wheat that my blood sugar was rising dangerously, it greatly improved once I cut out wheat. I did not think to get this checked in the years following, because I was not eating sugar and wheat (which converts to sugar/glucose in the body).

As it turns out, on the glycemic index chart of 1–100 (1 being that the food in question raises your blood sugar very little, and 100 being that it raises it dangerously), white rice flour is an 89. Wheat flour—whole wheat or white—is "only" 70. Anything over 50 is given a high rating, so even brown rice, at 50, is not much better. I was stunned to discover that my rice flour and gluten-free lifestyle was doing more damage to my blood sugar levels than the wheat flour had done, now that I was consuming the rice flour so liberally. Not to mention the fact that I ate so much fruit every day and I also juiced fruit (and vegetables) every single morning. My body was consuming so many carbs through this liquid, so many natural sugars, and all the rice products, that I wound up in a prediabetic state and became insulin resistant. While eating no wheat, sugar or junk! Ever! Once I limited my fruit and rice products and tried to stick to only 20–25 carbs each day, and I increased my healthy fats and proteins (with endless vegetables), my blood sugar quickly stabilized. As a nice side benefit, I also dropped ten pounds almost effortlessly. In less than a month. And another five in the next month, for a total of fifteen pounds. And I was full all the time.

So, if you are someone whom God has convicted to live a sugar-free, wheat-free lifestyle and you have seen miraculous improvements in your health (which you will, because those are both so hard on the body to process), maintain your miracle by not going overboard with everything labeled "gluten-free." And when you do need flour, consider nut flours instead: almond, walnut, coco"nut" and others. They contain a lot of protein, omega-3s, amino acids and vitamins. They help control your blood sugar because of the plant fiber and keep you full until the next meal.

Whenever I begin discussing life changes with people, there is always someone who chimes in with the "my aunt ate junk and lived to be 110" defense. We have all heard of these folks or have seen them on the news. My nutritionist tells me that people who live long despite poor health choices either (1) grew up with a garden and have incredible "reserves" to sustain their health, (2) have Native American in their blood, or (3) honored their mother and father. There is a definite truth to that last once since the fifth commandment is the first to end with a promise, telling us that if we honor our parents, we will live a long and happy life in the land God gives us. But the point is that we cannot dismiss the importance of personal responsibility just because a few people defy the statistics. Imagine how much longer the dietarily defiant could live with just some simple changes!

What are those simple changes? Well, when we practice the "Eight Laws of Health," a divine grace rests on our body to remain disease-free and vibrant. And what are these eight laws? They are principles Dr. Jim Sharps of IIOM promotes in his book *Concepts of Original Medicine*.[1] He says these eight laws are the foundational principles for experiencing outrageous health and vitality. I would like to outline them for you here with my own commentary, and a bit of his. Here are the eight things that are vital to vibrant health, or as Dr. Sharps calls it, "radiant health."

1. Pure Air

Sitting down to write this section on air, it dawned on me that I had not been outside in a couple of days for some fresh air. On my small patio I have a hammock that hangs from an arbor my husband built, and it is honestly the greatest enticement to get me outside and breathing deeply for my daily "air bath." As a writer, I spend a great amount of time indoors. Perhaps you work indoors, too. If so, surrounding you are chemicals, carbon dioxide, carbon monoxide and other pollutants.

In fact, the phrase "sick-building disease" (or "sick-building syndrome") originates from people in the last several generations noticing a decline in their overall health from breathing in carpet fibers, paint and other environmental toxins day after

1. See Dr. Jim Sharps, *Concepts of Original Medicine* (Smithfield, Virginia: International Institute of Original Medicine, 2013).

day for years. And this is not just the case in old, run-down buildings, because even new paint and chemicals can be toxic. Plus, most buildings not only contain these toxins; they are also sealed with manipulated ventilation (manmade filtering) that never allows the pollutants to be fully removed. As a result, you see an increase in allergies, infections, a worsening of asthma symptoms, depression and even Legionnaires' disease.

We cannot heal if we cannot breathe, and we cannot walk in vibrant health if we are not breathing pure air. It heals wounds, increases energy, purges the mind and seemingly purifies the soul with our deep breathing. It is obvious that air is the most important nutrient to humankind, as evidenced by the fact that the typical human cannot go more than three minutes without air and live. You can go without water for days and without food for weeks, but you can only go minutes without breathing.

How miraculous that God designed our bodies to breathe whether awake or asleep, conscious or unconscious. In fact, Dr. Sharps points out that you cannot even commit suicide by holding your breath, because at the point of passing out, the brain stem takes over and forces you to breathe again. Pure air is a gift from God, and we should plan ahead and practice the deep breathing of it in our daily routines.

2. Pure Water

Did you know that your body is 70 to 75 percent water? Amazingly, so is the planet. It is as if God has made your body a walking picture of the earth. Of course, that should be no wonder since He literally created man from the earth. But practically speaking, this means that a 140-pound woman houses about 100 pounds of water. This is also why consuming too much sodium, which retains water, can wreak such havoc on our weight.

Your muscles are made up of about 75 percent water, the brain's gray matter is approximately 85 percent water, and the blood is about 83 percent water. All the body's major processes require water, including cell reproduction, circulation, digestion, elimination and more. Pure water is a blessing to humans, animals and even all the earth's vegetation.

Make sure to drink ample healthy, filtered water daily. How much? This is a topic of great debate. As a simple rule, typically I recommend consuming half your body weight in ounces of water each day. But people who consistently eat a 50 percent raw vegetable diet (which is rare, unfortunately) get much of their water quota from their food and need not drown themselves in even more water, which ultimately just dilutes their digestive juices. Also to be considered are other lifestyle factors such as exercise (including how much one sweats) and caffeine-consumption (which is dehydrating). So alongside my recommendation to aim for eight glasses of water daily, there is a parenthetical option for you to drink four to five glasses if you are disciplined about your raw vegetable consumption.

3. Sunlight

If you want increased energy, energized blood and a healthy complexion, you can have it all for free just by stepping outside and enjoying the free vitamin D in the sky—the sun. A mere twenty minutes a day of sunshine can do amazing things for your body and mind. Let's look at a few.

For example, sunlight aids digestion and weight loss goals. Why? First, it unlocks vitamins in your food. You will find that with ample sunshine, you will crave less heavy food. Sunshine is good for reaching your weight goals.

Sunlight also has a positive effect on mood and emotional health. Sunshine brings a sense of peace, joy and contentment.

We all know that the weather affects our moods, even if we are indoors on a rainy day. Lack of sunlight during the winter months has been linked to seasonal affective disorder—aptly abbreviated SAD—causing many to purchase indoor sunlamps to avoid depression. How amazing is it that God has set in the sky such a free source of joy and happiness? (Both the sun and His Son!)

Sunlight even promotes healing. Your nerve endings actually absorb the transmitted energy from the sun, resulting in increased energy. Due to this increase in energy and the sun's ability to permeate the skin and control the chemistry of the blood, sunlight also expedites detoxification and healing. I remember discovering once as a young girl that my cold symptoms went away after a day in the summer sun. I had not wanted to tell my mother I felt sick, lest she keep me home, but after just a short while in the sun I was totally asymptomatic. Was it the pool water? (No, there was chlorine in it.) Was it the rest? (Probably not, since I was running around the pool and swimming vigorously.) By process of elimination, I learned over time that the common denominator was merely time in the healing sun. Just ten minutes in the midday sun with your arms and legs showing will activate about 10,000 international units (IU) of vitamin D, which is a key treatment for colds and flu, not to mention the prevention of them. Plus, the raising of the body's temperature in the sun creates a fake fever, causing bacteria and germs in your body to die out. If you are fair-skinned, as I am, you may be thinking of using sunscreen, but be aware that sunscreen will decrease your vitamin D activation. Depending on your skin tone, humans are safe for ten to twenty minutes in the sun without any sunscreen (ten minutes for fair skin and twenty minutes for darker). Do not go beyond that and put yourself at risk for skin cancer.

4. Good Nutrition

It goes without saying that healthy nutrition leads to health. You can literally change your life with your fork. Your car cannot run on the wrong kind of gas, and your body cannot run on the wrong kind of food, although I use the term *food* loosely here since much of what we consume today our bodies do not even recognize as food. In the words of Dr. Sharps in *Concepts of Original Medicine*,

> Fundamentally, the best foods for physical nourishment and health are living, whole foods as they were created by God and provided by nature. All the knowledge we have gained since the beginning of time continually supports this simple fact. Nature, in the form of plant foods, supplies all the food and medicine we need for physical health. Nature provides the most perfect food laboratory—one that yields an abundant menu of wholesome vitamins, minerals, proteins, carbohydrates, fats and other essential known and unknown nutrients. Fruits, vegetables, nuts, grains, seeds and edible herbs, properly prepared and in adequate amounts, supply all the nutrients required for developing and maintaining optimum health. Especially when eaten raw, the life of the food in the form of enzymes is still present and is highly beneficial to the body. This forms the basis of the dietary principles of original medicine.[2]

When people ask me why I decided to get a degree in Original Medicine, that paragraph provides my best answer. The A-list I provide you at the end of every body system blessing in part two will give you some nourishing advice for the system being prayed for—fruits, vegetables, spices and more. You will even learn which vitamins or supplements you should take and which essential oils to apply while focusing on that body system. If

2. Sharps, *Concepts of Original Medicine*, 42–43.

you are a meat eater, you will find some meat options, but I encourage you to experience the health surge of getting your protein from plant-based sources. Still, if you do eat meat, always choose antibiotic-free meat. If beef, choose hormone-free, grass fed. (Remember, "you are what you eat eats").

But whatever you consume, remember to chew each bite thirty times, mixing the food with saliva, which is the beginning of the digestive process. Those digestive juices are important, so give them a head start by savoring the smell of the food as you cook it and gratefully gather around the table to eat it. How amazing that when we stop and take the time to pray over our meal, it actually gives our digestive tract time to get prepared for its job.

If you will diligently adhere to each body system's A-list, and if you will apply these "Eight Laws of Health," you will have all the tools necessary to become a better and more vibrant you.

5. Exercise

Dr. Sharps also makes the noteworthy point that our entire universe is set up around the principle of movement. He explains that if anything quits moving—the sun, moon, stars, rivers, clouds—everything is altered and all life ceases to exist. It should be no surprise, therefore, that it is the same with our bodies. Movement engages all your major body systems, from your cardiovascular system to your muscular system, to your nervous system, to your skeletal system, lymphatic system and more. In death, all these systems cease their movement entirely. So shouldn't it make sense that if you want to live now, your life must include movement?

Our bodies were made to move. It is easier to move for thirty minutes than to stand still for thirty minutes, proving that movement is necessary for optimum physical and mental health. Exercise lowers blood pressure, strengthens bones, promotes good cholesterol, wards off cancer, decreases depression tendencies, improves posture and is an important part of controlling and preventing diabetes. Find your favorite way to move and start moving! Dancing, walking, running, biking, gardening, aerobics, Pilates, dog walking and yes, even cleaning house burns calories and promotes movement.

Exercise does not come naturally to me. I have never been athletic or found any particular sport that could hold my interest long enough to keep me committed. That, coupled with being a writer, means a very sedentary lifestyle for me. When I was younger I was chasing six children everywhere, but now I have to be more intentional about movement. It seems I am always writing or editing what I wrote, or creating and editing a video to market what I just wrote. All of those involve sitting. Even going to one of my own book signings results in . . . more sitting. And what do I do when counseling people at our church? Sit. And what do we do *in* church? Sit. (Thank goodness for our exuberant worship beforehand at Eastgate.) All things put together, I am a pretty stationary gal. I have never had a serious weight issue, but all of that sitting with a slowing metabolism is not good. Last year I decided to force myself into movement, so I bought an exercise bike desk. Yep! Since I have no desk at my house (by choice), if I want to write, I now have a vow with myself that I will do it on this exercise bike desk. I used to plop on the sofa to write or jump on our fluffy bed with my laptop and spend hours writing. Now, I do not let myself do that. In fact, I am writing this entire book on my exercise bike desk. (The Exerpeutic WorkFit 1000 Fully Adjustable Desk Folding Exercise Bike with Pulse, in case you are wondering.)

You should have seen my face when I first saw the bicycle that Chosen's design team put on the front cover of this book, with its tires making up the double *O* in *SOON*. At first I did not want the bicycle there, because I felt we needed a symbol for the mind. I had asked for some of the title's letters to be images, and since my branding is that of a body, mind and spirit author, I had suggested the praying/healing hands for the *W* in *WELL*, and the carrot for the *T* in *GET*. I was hoping the design team could come up with a symbol for one of the letters in *SOON* that would represent the mind. If the carrot was food for the body and the hands were food for the spirit, I felt we needed a symbol more representative of the mind than the bike at first seemed to be. But the more I thought about it, the more I realized that the bike was like a "God-wink" affirming the commitment I have made to move more on this desk bike as I put my mind to work writing books. But it also means that it is a message God wants me to communicate to *you* so you can get well soon: You must start moving!

At present, I have cycled 62.9 miles while writing this book. Check back at the end of the book to see my final mileage. I also still have my trusty portable treadmill in my bedroom for quick runs, the same one I mentioned in *The Healthy Living Handbook* (the Confidence Power Plus Motorized Fitness Treadmill). Its off-white color matches my bedroom; therefore, it can stay there and stare me down each day. I find that if you just hop on with your phone and check your social media sites, before you know it you have run a mile. Ask the Lord for your own exercise strategy and He will surely give it to you, as He did to me.

6. Adequate Rest

I have already shared with you how lack of sleep almost cost me my life in my late forties. If you do not go to sleep, your organs will go to sleep for you. They must rejuvenate, and that only happens at night when you sleep. Psalm 127:2 tells us that God gives His beloved sleep. Of course, He gives us many other things that we do not take advantage of, such as spiritual gifts, healing, love and even salvation. So sleep is not automatic, either, and often we must fight for it.

Nighttime is a sacred time. As I explained in my book *Seeing the Voice of God: What God is Telling You through Dreams & Visions* (Chosen, 2014), God did not create the moon, stars and nighttime as an afterthought during the creation process. He designed these special hours of each day as a time for us to rest, even turning out the lights for us so that we might sleep even better. You see, when light hits our optic nerve, it signals our pineal gland that it is time to wake up. So this gland shuts down its production of melatonin, which is "the drowsy hormone." This is why leaving the light off when you get up in the middle of the night to go to the bathroom is so vital to getting back to sleep, as is limiting your use of electronics just before bedtime if you want to fall asleep faster. People who say they need the TV on to fall asleep do not realize that their bodies are not fully entering into a deep rest, because that light constantly is sending the message to their optic nerve and pineal gland that it is time to wake up. You may fall asleep out of utter exhaustion with the TV on, but it would be healthier (and more peaceful) to find another way to fall asleep.

I give plenty of suggestions about sleep in chapter 4 of *Seeing the Voice of God*, under "Laura's ABCs for ZZZs Sleep Tips." Chapters 4 and 5 are dedicated to the improvement of your sleep through very specific wind-down steps you take as you are downshifting into sleep each night, and also to the vitamins and minerals you can take to improve your dream recall. It is a book about how our multitasking God desires to connect with us through the precious hours of the night, speaking direction to us that will help us make better decisions when awake.

Not to mention that we must sleep, period, which many people cannot do. They are in a war with the enemy himself to take back their ability to get to sleep or stay asleep. It is yet another reason why I created my Quiet Brain essential oil blend (more about that in chapter 10, but you can also go to quietbrainoil.com). I am happy to say that it is helping countless people all over the world accomplish getting a full night's rest. If I could put a bottle of Quiet Brain oil and a copy of *Seeing the Voice of God* in everyone's hand in the world, I would! But with the billions of people on this earth, that would cost $587,650,000,000! But I know that God has given me keys to help others sleep better, longer, with more peace and with better ability to remember their dreams. Better sleep health leads to overall improved health, so if your health is bad, begin by examining your sleep health. Do whatever you must do (within the realm of what is healthy) to get adequate sleep each night, and watch everything about you change. Your body's ability to heal will change (through the release of the human growth hormone as you sleep), along with your complexion (they don't call it beauty rest for nothing), your weight (sleep helps balance cortisol during stress, which, if unbalanced, leads to belly fat), your moods (nothing like sleep deprivation to give you a case of the grumpies), and even your outlook about your future.

Sleep is not an afterthought in the design of your body. It is essential to its health. Even God Himself rested after creation was complete. Exodus 20:8–10 tells us,

> Remember the Sabbath day, to keep it holy. Six days you shall labor, and do all your work, but the seventh day is a Sabbath to the LORD your God. On it you shall not do any work, you, or your son, or your daughter, your male servant, or your female servant, or your livestock, or the sojourner who is within your gates.

Our God commands us to rest and sets an example for us. If He can do it, so can you.

7. Temperance

Another word for temperance is *moderation*. The problem with the phrase "all things in moderation" is that people have different meanings for the word *moderation*. Some might perceive this to mean that they can partake of a small amount of something every now and again. Some others might define moderation as enjoying a little bit of something every single day. Still others might say that they can have too much of something, as long as they only do it occasionally. Countless times, I have actually heard people use the phrase "all things in moderation" and say it is in the Bible, quoting it as if it has the authority of Scripture. But the Bible would never say "all things" in moderation, for certainly murder in moderation is not acceptable, nor is adultery, lying, pornography, premarital sex, physical abuse, etc. People get this phrase either from the Greek poet Hesiod (circa 700 BC), who said, "Observe due measure; moderation is best in all things," or from the Roman comic dramatist Plautus (circa 254–184 BC), who said, "Moderation in all things is the best policy."

This misguided phrase basically gives you a blank check to do whatever you feel like doing at least some of the time, which I think is unscriptural. So I like Dr. Sharps's choice of the word *temperance* over *moderation*. It is a Middle English word from the Anglo-Norman French *temperaunce*, and also from Latin's *temperare*, meaning "restrain." In English it means "abstinence from alcoholic drink,"[3] and you may be familiar with the temperance movement of the nineteenth century, which began around the 1820s and advocated total abstinence from alcohol. This movement was successful in lowering national crime rates, but the laws of total prohibition (making both the consumption of and resale of liquor illegal) did not last

3. *English Oxford Living Dictionaries*, s.v. "Temperance," accessed July 16, 2018, https://en.oxforddictionaries.com/definition/temperance.

long, because prohibition also lowered national revenues, city by city.

Of course, this section is about restraint in many more things besides just alcohol. We must also exercise restraint—or self-control—at all times in all things. God tells us in Galatians 5 that having self-control is actually an indicator of having the Holy Spirit. It is a fruit of His Spirit; the fruit of truly having *Him*.

It does seem that in each of my books, the topic of alcohol winds up edging its way into the conversation. I never (ever) intend to discuss it, never have it in my outline, and, in fact, prefer not to discuss it due to the sharp division it causes. Yet when I am addressing health as a nutritionist, alcohol cannot help but creep into the conversation in this day and age. So many people are wondering what is permissible in the spiritual concerning it, and even if they are sure of having the Spirit's permission, they question what is profitable for the body. It is for the sake of these very questions that I created an e-book on the topic that I prefer to refer people to when they are inquiring about this stiff debate over temperance. You can download it for free on my website (lauraharrissmith.com/ebooks). Called *Wine & Spirits*, it is an unbiased book about three very biased characters: the Prohibitionist, the Moderationist and the Abstentionist.[4] The book is full of Scripture, science and statistics, and at the end of each informative chapter, the three characters process their opinions about it all, leaving you equipped to form your own opinion. You are welcome to enjoy it and see what the Lord speaks to you on this topic. For many, alcohol falls into a category they call "awful but lawful," while many others contend that it is not lawful at all, and many more will insist that there is not the slightest thing awful about.

4. Laura Harris Smith, *Wine & Spirits: A Balanced Christian Commentary on the Christian's Choice to Drink*, LHS Ministries, 2016, https://view.publitas.com/laura-harris-smith-ministries/wine-spirits-e-book/page/1.

Wherever you land, please remember that the topic of temperance itself extends far beyond this "little" discussion over alcohol. Temperance is a lifestyle. Avoid any health-destroying habits in your life, whether they involve behaviors, foods, thoughts, drink or relationships. Even ask the Lord to help you to discern how to act wisely about the less controversial items on your list, such as junk food, nicotine, caffeine, the overuse of prescription drugs and even workaholism. We must choose between better and best, between permissible and profitable.

Romans 12:2 tells us, "And be not conformed to this world: but be ye transformed by the renewing of your mind, that ye may prove what is that good, and acceptable, and perfect, will of God" (KJV). I believe this shows that there is a good will of God, an acceptable will of God, and a perfect will of God. In other words, for your life He has a good will, an acceptable will, and a perfect will. Of course, He would prefer that you abide by His perfect will, but sometimes it is just not possible. One example would be that God says in His Word that He hates divorce (see Malachi 2:16), yet if your spouse files against your will, God's perfect will cannot be accomplished in the marriage any longer. For you, that divorce becomes God's acceptable will for your life.

In this area of temperance and self-control, ask God to show you His perfect will. Not just what is good or acceptable, but perfect. Just be brave and ask. I believe every believer goes through three stages in learning what is God's will for his or her life. Early on, new Christians assume anything is permissible because of God's grace, and they settle for less than perfect. Then maybe they begin maturing in greater measures of consecration and holiness, but they still make compromises, opting merely for what is acceptable. But for those who seek God in the minutia of their life, He will meet them with big answers.

I believe Mark 4, the parable of the sower, confirms this "three" teaching on God's will. It is a story in which all the characters finally planted in good soil with good seed, yet some yielded 30-fold returns, some 60-fold and some 100-fold. I have always wondered why that is. Have you noticed Christians around you who just seem content with obeying God 30 percent of the time, or maybe even 60 percent? I have. Well, I want to be a 100-fold, perfect-will-of-God Christian. I am not interested in a 30-fold "acceptable" life, or a 60-fold "good" life. I may not hit the 100-fold, perfect-will-of-God mark every time, but it will not be said of Laura Harris Smith that she did not try with all her might.

8. Trust in Divine Power

Dr. Jim Sharps said, "Of all the eight laws of natural health, this law should be the most sacredly cherished because our every breath, good health, and the essence of all healing come from the Creator."[5] I agree with him entirely. Every word of this book you are reading is intended to bring you closer to your Creator, so I will let the rest of it now speak to you about your trust in God as your Great Physician. That connection is paramount if you are to be healthy physically, emotionally and spiritually. Of what good is perfect physical health without a healthy spirit? None, for the physical health you work so hard to achieve will fade without wisdom whispered from the Holy Spirit on what to incorporate and exclude from your daily life—not to mention the fact that the body fades, but the spirit is eternal. If you will practice the very basic steps of connecting with God daily through time in His Word, listening prayer and loving your neighbor, you will tap into divinely empowered living. And here are some parting words of wisdom from Dr. Sharps:

> Spiritual health keeps our entire being in balance. It provides the healthy soil that brings forth good fruit. It prevents us from

5. Sharps, *Concepts of Original Medicine*, 52.

being overweight and overbearing. Just as fruit and vegetables are the staples for supporting our physical health, unconditional love and forgiveness are the primary staples for supporting spiritual health. Peace, joy, humility, and wisdom are the nuts, seeds, grains, and legumes that round out a complete whole-food diet that supports our spiritual health.[6]

In case you have not noticed, this is the longest chapter of any so far in this book. I suppose the reason is that I am *determined* to help you maintain the miracles you are going to receive and the healings you are going to set into motion in part two.

Now that you have decided just how well you want to be, have taken inventory of your health, have acknowledged that God did not make you sick, have discovered the root of your condition, have learned how to pray the prayer of faith, have prepared yourself for the unleashing of the blessing and the reversing of the curse, have learned how to watch your words and have discovered how to maintain your miracle, it is time to learn the difference between a healing and a miracle—a revelation that changed my life and health forever.

6. Ibid., 55.

9

Know the Difference between Healings and Miracles

I t took me years to believe in healing in the first place. Twenty-five years, in fact. Growing up in church I never heard about miracles or healings, not even when I was diagnosed with epilepsy at thirteen years old. It was not that we did not believe they could happen. It was more like I did not know if they would, or if God wanted them to happen at all. I had led Bible studies from the time I was thirteen, so I had plenty of opportunity to find the healing Scriptures for myself, but perhaps I had felt no urgent need to. But now here I was, as a young mother of twenty-nine, and Scriptures were suddenly becoming illuminated to me that I had overlooked after all those years of reading, learning and teaching the Bible. This coincided with increasing ailments that left me desperate for healing, and it took three long years for God to convince me that not only *could* He heal me, but that He also *would*.

I tell the full story in chapter 9 of *Seeing the Voice of God*, and I urge you to read it because countless people have told me it ministered to them in a profound way. It was during this time that I had a powerful encounter with God in my living room, in which He settled the issue once and for all for me. The date was January 26, 1993. I would call it a visitation from Him, because one minute I was merely kneeling and reading my Bible, and the next minute I was keenly aware of the fact that a King had come for a visit. A holy hush fell over the entire room, and every moment got big. I literally fell over—gently but swiftly—onto my face, unable to move. I feared that if I even looked up at Him, my flesh would melt off my whole body. But I was not afraid. He had not come so that I could look at Him. He had come to answer the question He knew my heart had been asking for months: *God, do You really want to heal me?*

His answer? He said He had already begun to heal me, but that it would be "by process." It has indeed been a twenty-plus-year process now of gradual improvement. On a healing scale of 1–10, with 10 being totally healed and 1 being the horrible neurological condition I once lived in, I would say I am now about a 9.5. And most days, a 10! At 53 years of age, I feel better than ever before in my life, and along the way I have become the me who is able to minister to you. I could not have become that minister any other way.

You cannot help but put emphasis on dramatic encounters like mine, but it needs to be said that even if the King of kings does not visit you personally to promise healing in the same way He visited me, you already have His promise in His Word. Visit with Him every day in your favorite healing Scriptures, from Genesis to Revelation. He is your Healer. So why does healing sometimes come late, or seemingly not at all?

That was a huge source of discouragement to me at one time. In fact, the hardest part of my "by process" healing was surprisingly not the physical symptoms that were in my body, but the psychological warfare in my mind. The enemy was telling me constantly that God had not promised me healing. That I had misunderstood Him. That I had misinterpreted Scripture. That I would never be well. What was equally discouraging was when people I loved and trusted seemed to agree with the devil and go out of their way to tell me so, in so many words. To tell me I had misunderstood God. To tell me I was misinterpreting Scripture. To tell me I probably would not be healed.

With friends and family like that, who needs enemies? I will not name names, but it was awful and occasionally vicious. It would emotionally set me back days at a time, doubting myself and doubting that God was who Scripture said He was. But eventually, the discouragement was only for hours, then minutes, and then seconds. And now, I can tell you with total honesty that I am totally immune to the enemy's discouragements. No matter if they come from Satan himself or out of the mouth of someone I love. It rolls right off me as if it had never been spoken. At the very most, the only emotion I feel is pity for the one who is working so hard to disprove God's Word. Doubters will doubt and naysayers will always say nay, but those who endure to the end will be saved and delivered, not to mention be spared from the negative, miserable mentality that the doubters suffer from! Besides, people have marked my progress all these years and have seen what God has done for me, so all the naysayers and doubters are gone. I simply cannot find one anywhere anymore.

Has God ever required you to wait on a healing—body, mind or spirit? If so, I am about to tell you something you may have overlooked in Scripture. I certainly had. It is hidden in 1 Corinthians 12, in a list of nine spiritual gifts available to us as believers. Even long after I welcomed each gift into my life one by one, I never realized that I had been merging two of the gifts together, as if they were one gift. Let's look at the list from verses 8–10:

1. word of wisdom
2. word of knowledge
3. faith
4. gifts of healing
5. the working of miracles
6. prophecy
7. discerning of spirits
8. speaking in tongues
9. interpretation of tongues

Suddenly, gifts number 4 and 5 jumped out at me—healing and miracles. Why were they listed as two different gifts? Were not healing and miracles both instant manifestations? But then it hit me: If God had intended for healing and miracles to be the same thing, then He would have named only eight spiritual gifts. The two were different somehow, and I had to figure out why. I then noticed in verse 28 that He distinguished them once more: "And God has appointed in the church first apostles, second prophets, third teachers, then miracles, then gifts of healing, helping, administrating, and various kinds of tongues."

There it was again—an undeniable mention of miracles and healings as two separate spiritual encounters. I suddenly knew I had to go to the Greek to figure out what these two words even meant. I was shocked that the meanings were not at all what I had thought. Let's first look at the various Greek words[1] for *miracle*:

1. All Greek word definitions here are taken from Blue Letter Bible's lexicon at https://www.blueletterbible.org.

dynamis—"strength power, force, might, energy, physical power; the abstract for the concrete." Also, it means "inherent power, power residing in a thing by virtue of its nature, or which a person or thing exerts and puts forth, the power for performing miracles, power consisting in or resting upon armies, forces, hosts."

The first definition of *dynamis* implies that something very tangible materialized from something intangible. The second definition implies a "power" word; the word *dynamite* has its origin here.

sēmeion—yet another Greek word meaning "miracle," as in "a sign; a mark; a token; unusual occurrence, transcending the common course of nature; of signs portending remarkable events soon to happen; miracles and wonders by which God authenticates the men sent by him, or by which men prove that the cause they are pleading is God's."

In other words, according to the definition of *sēmeion*, a miracle is an immediate sign that occurs seemingly to validate the one preaching the Gospel to others, to prove that God is in their midst. *Sēmeion* is very obviously a *"now"* word.

Together, these Greek definitions of *miracle* seem to convey "power *now*!" But what about *healing*? Is it a "power *now*!" word? No, it is not. In fact, look at these multiple Greek definitions for *healing* and notice how they are different from the previous two "power *now*!" words:

therapeuo or *therapeia*—"a service rendered, specifically a medical service"

kalos—"to be well and recover"

lama—"medicine; remedy; a means of healing," from *laomai*, meaning "to cure or heal"

The first word, *therapeuo* (or *therapeia*), is where we get the word *therapy*; thus, it is a "process" word. The second word, *kalos*, is found in Mark 16:18 (emphasis added): "They will lay their hands on the sick, and they will *recover*." *Recovery*, too, is a "process" word. The third word, *iama*, is another "process" word. Medicine, remedies and cures take time. Wouldn't you agree?

Have you noted yet that healings and miracles are *not* the same thing? They are as different as night and day. Miracles are immediate, and healings are progressive. But both are equally spectacular. And evidently, God Himself decides which one is best for you. But why would He do that? Why would He not want you to have everything *now*?

If you have a child (or have ever been one), you know the answer to that! Children want everything right now. ("Are we there yet?") But it is in the waiting that bigger and better things can manifest. During the waiting, God is able to work *all* things together for our good. Not just some. Do you want some, or all, of what God has for you? I want it all. But *all* takes longer than *some*. And a lot of the *somes* quit just before the *alls* come. Never settle for *some*!

So if you prayed for a miracle and it did not come immediately, perhaps God saw fit to give you a healing instead. But you should still rejoice, even if you are in process! You should never walk away dejectedly, saying, "I didn't get my miracle." No, you should rejoice and tell everyone that God saw fit to heal you instead. Then you can explain that this means you are now in a process of recovery. Healings do not happen at altars.

You may be thinking, *What, Laura?!* Here is what I mean by that: You cannot go through a "by process" therapy or medical recovery progression at an altar, since the Bible indicates that the word *healing* is a process. Likewise, if you experienced an immediate manifestation of physical relief at an altar, you did not get a healing. You got a miracle. But to say that one is better than the other is wrong. That is like saying that one of God's Galatians 5 fruits of the Spirit is better than the others, or one of God's prophets is better than the others, or even one of His kids is better than another! We have to trust whatever God gives us. In fact, the spiritual gifts list in 1 Corinthians 12:11 (NIV) actually ends by stating, "All these are the work of one and the same Spirit, and he distributes them to each one, just as he determines."

So God Himself decides if you are going to receive a healing or a miracle. And getting a healing is nothing to be ashamed of. It does not always mean that you do not have enough faith, but instead means that God has something even better and deeper in mind for you. It often means He wants you to focus on your spirit and mind being made whole, as well as your body, whereas with a bodily miracle it is often easy to forget the other two-thirds of your being and never deal with them. I always say that healings are an invitation. I practically have this concept memorized because I recite it all the time: "Walk with Me. Trust Me. Rest in Me and recover with Me. Let *Me* be your cure and therapy." I am constantly shocked at how many people have overlooked this special gift in Scripture of a progressive healing. It is a process.

There are so many more definitions in Scripture we could turn to for the word *healing*. In fact, it could be one of nine Greek words or fourteen Hebrew words, and each one gives insight into this beautiful gift called wellness. Healings are not second-class answers to prayer. They just mean you are in the middle of a miracle, so to speak.

This is how 1 Corinthians 12:9–10 would read with the Greek definitions inserted: "To some I have given the ability to work instant miracles and to others I have given the ability to invent, discover and provide God's cures and medicines." When you pray for a miracle in your body, mind or spirit and you do not see it manifest immediately, praise God for all to hear and say, "I got my healing!" Maybe that seems fake to you. But what it means is that you are in a recovery process with the Great Physician, and that He has greater things in store for you than you originally asked or imagined. It means that the process will bring a thorough healing to your mind and spirit, too.

Now that you have decided just how well you want to be, taken inventory of your health, acknowledged that God did not make you sick, discovered the root of your condition, learned how to pray the prayer of faith, prepared yourself for the unleashing of the blessing and the reversing of the curse, learned how to watch your words, discovered how to maintain your miracle and understood the difference between a healing and a miracle, it is time for you to learn to love the you that you are becoming. This is a book of change. Prepare yourself for the new you!

10

Love the You
You're Becoming

Sometimes, you do *everything* Scripture says, yet healing is delayed. You learn a lot about yourself during these times. I shared with you how God told me during that January 1993 visitation that He was going to heal me "by process." This route was not the miracle I had total and unswerving faith for, so it made no sense to me why I could not attain it immediately. But in the waiting, I grew in Him. I grew in prayer. I had to learn the healing Scriptures enough to cling to them, not to mention defend them to the naysayers.

It was also during this discouraging phase that I became an encourager. I felt the best way I could give the devil a black eye during these "Dark Ages of Discouragement" was to encourage others the way I desperately needed to be encouraged. I used to go to Christian gatherings and meetings and think, *If only someone would give me a word of encouragement while I am here. If only God would tell me through someone that He is with me and has not forgotten me.* It would have been life to me!

One day, I just decided to become that person of encouragement for others. I felt so powerful against my enemy, more powerful than I had ever felt before in my life. I had the power to wipe away whatever bad day, week or month Satan had tried to lay on someone. I could, by God's grace, change the entire atmosphere of a person's day or a life by just making my mouth available to God. I developed an eagle eye for being able to walk into a room and detect who needed encouraging. I would ask God for prophetic words for them, and the words would flow. Tears would come, laughter would follow, and I would leave feeling energized. I even began not to need encouragement myself anymore, because my deepest question about God being with me was being answered. He obviously was with me, as evidenced by the accurate prophetic words I was getting for people. Out of my deepest days of despair came some of the most accurate prophecies about unborn babies (who were born), troubled marriages (which were restored), financial breakthroughs (one guy even won the lottery), and of course physical healing. I was not even a pastor at the time. I was just a woman who knew what it was like to be discouraged, and who decided not to let others around me have to experience that. Years later, I looked around me and had an army of encouragers who were cheering me on, as well. We definitely reap what we sow. I think that is a major reason God made my healing "by process"—because I needed those traits for the ministry I am in today, as both a pastor and a public speaker.

In the meantime, though, I had to figure out ways to stay healthy (even stay alive) while I waited on God. This led to my original interest in nutrition in the mid-1990s. When I seemed to get worse over the next ten years—not better, as promised—it made me press in even harder to prayer and research. From the time I first began to investigate nutrition in 1993, until I began to lean on it entirely twenty years later, in 2013, I learned more than I could ever have imagined. Earning my nutritionist certification and my bachelor's and master's degrees in Original Medicine after that was *nothing* in comparison to those first painful twenty years, mainly because I was in the neurological fight for my life during that earlier time.

Would God have let me perish if I had lain around and done nothing during my "process" recovery? That is a good question, but I think the answer is no. It was not enough, however, for me barely to escape death. I wanted to thrive. And while learning to thrive, I woke up one day and realized I had a blossoming ministry of helping others thrive. I was learning to comfort others with the comfort with which I had been comforted (see 2 Corinthians 1:4).

But it was not until 2016 that I saw perhaps the most significant reason why God had chosen a healing for me and not a miracle. My healing seemed almost complete, and I had never felt neurologically healthier. Still, if I stayed up too late or let myself get overworked and sleep deprived, I would have some smaller episodes of what are called "breakthrough seizures." They only affected my concentration, and no one knew but me that I had experienced one. They were quicker than a sneeze, but a definite break in consciousness. And if these misfires happened often enough within a short time frame, a massive headache would follow. It was obvious to me that I was not at the end of my "by process" recovery, so I dug in deeper.

I had never ventured far into the land of essential oils, because, honestly, I could not find single oils that did much neurologically for me. I had quite an arsenal of them for more minor things like colds, flu and tummy aches, and whenever I would hear of a single oil that would help with brain issues, I would try it. But one oil just did not seem to help me on its own. Then one day, my oldest adult son told me that just one drop of cedarwood helped him sleep. I had to do some research and figure out if this was even plausible.

It certainly was. It turns out cedarwood oil is comprised of a special compound made up of sesquiterpenes, and these are actually able to cross the blood-brain barrier (BBB). The brain has its own security system—and how miraculous that it does, or else things you eat or drink might find their way to it and seep through. But it is that security barrier that also keeps many medications out of the brain, which is not a good thing if your brain is the organ that needs medication (as mine was). This explained the lifetime of seizures with no real relief from medications, and more doctors than I can count apologizing to me for being unable to help me. According to the American Society for Experimental Neurotherapeutics, researchers have even found that out of all the drugs for brain-related issues (neurological and mental), 98 percent of all small molecule drugs and 100 percent of all large molecule drugs cannot even pass through the BBB.[1] This means that millions upon millions of people suffering with neurological or mental issues are taking medications that may not even be getting to their brains. But the molecules in sesquiterpenes are so tiny that they *do pass through.* And because they are so tiny, our nasal passages can detect them. The oils that contain them are among the most aromatic of all oils.

The fact that cedarwood is comprised of 98 percent sesquiterpenes explains its potency. And now I was curious about whether there were other sesquiterpenes out there that were equally nourishing for the brain. What if I could create something that would help my own brain? What if it could help others? What if it could help my son-in-law, who had returned from two deployments in Iraq with a relentless case of PTSD? I set out on a quest to discover the most potent sesquiterpene essential oils that are brain nourishing, and I found eight, one of which was cedarwood. I ordered these eight costly oils and just stared at them for a month. I would take pictures of the bottles all lined up together, as if they were going to be something great, but then put them back in their box and wait for inspiration.

---

1. William M. Pardridge, "The Blood-Brain Barrier: Bottleneck in Brain Drug Development," National Center for Biotechnology Information, January 2005, http://www.ncbi.nlm.nih.gov/pmc/articles/PMC539316/.

Finally, one night it came. With all the children gone and my husband tucked away in his office, I got out the bottles again and sat down at my kitchen table. I turned on some worship music, opened the bottles and just waited. Five drops of this, ten drops of that, thirty of this, and then five more of the other. With a little pipette eyedropper I filled the very first bottle of Quiet Brain ever, keeping good notes of the final recipe on my phone. I suddenly became very aware of the presence of the Lord. It was so undeniable that I began to weep and just worship. I thanked God in advance for whatever it was that He had just accomplished.

When I was done, I screwed on the cap and just stared at the little bottle. Something was missing, but what? The bottle was full and the recipe complete, as inspired by the Holy Spirit. And then it dawned on me: The final ingredient was prayer.

I ran out to my husband's office—still crying—and told him what had just happened. I was overcome with God's presence and the "knowing" that something big was being birthed. "We have to pray over this and ask God to transform it into an anointing oil."

That is exactly what we did, and exactly what God did. Quiet Brain® was born.

I then felt impressed to do a case study, which meant I had to make more oil and I also had to keep everything safe. I went to the U.S. Food and Drug Administration's website and downloaded the appropriate forms that people need to sign when they participate in a case study. I gave explicit instructions to the participants on the application, after which they had to answer several questions such as what their symptoms were, whether or not the Quiet Brain helped relieve those symptoms, and if so, how quickly. I was not surprised when the testimonies began rolling in, because I knew I had something special, as evidenced by the presence of the Lord guiding me through the recipe. But I was very, very humbled. The case study evidenced relief from insomnia, migraines, tremors, seizures, anxiety, and yes, even my son-in-law's PTSD, as well as my occasional breakthrough seizures. Day or night, anytime I would experience the pesky misfirings, I would apply Quiet Brain to the top of my brain stem (the upper back of the neck, just under the hairline), and they would stop. Entirely. And instantly.

With the testimonies still flooding in, I felt led by the Lord to go through the trademarking process with the United States Patent and Trademark Office (USPTO). To do this, I had to show proof of commerce, which forced me to create a website for the oil: quietbrainoil.com. Soon after that, we entered into the patenting process with the USPTO to legally protect the recipe. Now, just two and a half years later, Quiet Brain is the largest selling item on our website (lauraharrissmith.com). It also plays a huge part in funding my television show, *theTHREE*, so named because of how each of us is comprised of three miraculous parts—body, mind and spirit—in the image of the miraculous Trinity.

Do you see my point? *All of this came from my suffering. All of this came from waiting. From pressing in. From persistence, research and total dependency on God.* If I had received a miracle in 1993 and not a "by process" healing, there would be no Quiet Brain, I would not be a nutritionist, and countless people in whom God wanted to do a deeper work of a progressive healing would not be receiving help from my ministry. You would not even be reading this book.

During the late nineties, a friend at our church, Carol Hanson, noticed that I was getting discouraged and absolutely consumed with the topic of God healing me. It was all I talked about, to the neglect of other things in my life, like patience. To me this focus felt obedient, faith-filled and exciting. But one day, Carol sent me an email with a word from the Lord. When I opened the email, it was not the prophetic word I wanted. Yet the creative way in which Carol delivered it drove home the Lord's point. It said,

Keep an eternal perspective. Keep an eternal perspective.
Keep an eternal perspective. Keep an eternal perspective.
Keep an eternal perspective. Keep an eternal perspective.
Keep an eternal perspective. Keep an eternal perspective.
Keep an eternal perspective. Keep an eternal perspective.
Keep an eternal perspective. Keep an eternal perspective.
Keep an eternal perspective. Keep an eternal perspective.
Keep an eternal perspective. Keep an eternal perspective.
Keep an eternal perspective. Keep an eternal perspective.
Keep an eternal perspective. Keep an eternal perspective.
Keep an eternal perspective. Keep an eternal perspective.
Keep an eternal perspective. Keep an eternal perspective.
Keep an eternal perspective. Keep an eternal perspective.
Keep an eternal perspective. Keep an eternal perspective.
Keep an eternal perspective. Keep an eternal perspective.
Keep an eternal perspective. Keep an eternal perspective.
Keep an eternal perspective. Keep an eternal perspective.
Keep an eternal perspective. Keep an eternal perspective.
Keep an eternal perspective. Keep an eternal perspective.
Keep an eternal perspective. Keep an eternal perspective.
Keep an eternal perspective. Keep an eternal perspective.
Keep an eternal perspective. Keep an eternal perspective.
Keep an eternal perspective. Keep an eternal perspective.
Keep an eternal perspective. Keep an eternal perspective.
Keep an eternal perspective. Keep an eternal perspective.
Keep an eternal perspective. Keep an eternal perspective.
Keep an eternal perspective. Keep an eternal perspective.

Keep an eternal perspective. Keep an eternal perspective.
Keep an eternal perspective. Keep an eternal perspective.
Keep an eternal perspective. Keep an eternal perspective.
Keep an eternal perspective. Keep an eternal perspective.
Keep an eternal perspective. Keep an eternal perspective.
Keep an eternal perspective. Keep an eternal perspective.
Keep an eternal perspective. Keep an eternal perspective.
Keep an eternal perspective. Keep an eternal perspective.
Keep an eternal perspective. Keep an eternal perspective.
Keep an eternal perspective. Keep an eternal perspective.
Keep an eternal perspective. Keep an eternal perspective.
Keep an eternal perspective. Keep an eternal perspective.
Keep an eternal perspective. Keep an eternal perspective.
Keep an eternal perspective. Keep an eternal perspective.
Keep an eternal perspective. Keep an eternal perspective.
Keep an eternal perspective. Keep an eternal perspective.
Keep an eternal perspective. Keep an eternal perspective.
Keep an eternal perspective. Keep an eternal perspective.
Keep an eternal perspective. Keep an eternal perspective.
Keep an eternal perspective. Keep an eternal perspective.
Keep an eternal perspective. Keep an eternal perspective.
Keep an eternal perspective. Keep an eternal perspective.
Keep an eternal perspective. Keep an eternal perspective.
Keep an eternal perspective. Keep an eternal perspective.
Keep an eternal perspective. Keep an eternal perspective.
Keep an eternal perspective. Keep an eternal perspective.

As I scrolled and scrolled down that email, I knew what God was trying to tell me through this visual word. He had more in mind for me than just a miracle. He wanted to give me a healing ministry that would bear Him much more eternal fruit, but it was going to require an investment, and investments take time. Today, I have that healing ministry, and part of it now extends to you. You are the fruit of my suffering. You are the reward for Jesus' suffering. Thank you for launching your journey toward health and for inviting me to be part of it. I am praying for you. Keep an eternal perspective.

Now that you have decided just how well you want to be, have taken inventory of your health, have acknowledged that God did not make you sick, have discovered the root of your condition, have learned how to pray the prayer of faith, have prepared yourself for the unleashing of the blessing and the reversing of the curse, have learned how to watch your words, have discovered how to maintain your miracle, have understood the difference between a healing and a miracle and have prepared yourself to meet (and love) the new you, you are in the most prime position of your life for change that bears lasting fruit in your body, mind and spirit. This, my friend, is the only path to being *whole*. It is the only path to *staying* whole.

In part two, we are going to bless each of your body systems and pray healing prayers against any disease that is invading them. But before that, you will read a declaration over each system to remind yourself of these ten steps you just learned, so that you can create an airtight, leakproof environment for breakthrough.

The things you have discovered and done in part one of this book have given you the blank canvas you need to get well soon. Are you now ready to paint miracles and healing on it in part two?

Blessings and Healing Prayers for Your Whole Body

wrote the 15 body system blessings and 200-plus healing prayers in this part of the book for you with prayerful fasting, and I invite you to partake of them with the same investment. Pray them in an unrushed, quiet environment, and consider using worship music to tune your spirit to the Holy Spirit before you start. I would also like to speak these blessings over you myself, so visit lauraharrissmith.com/blessings to see and hear me do that for you via video.

To build your faith, I have also included testimonies in each chapter that come from men and women who have experienced dramatic healings and miracles after praying these same exact prayers you are about to pray and reading the very blessings you are about to read. Some of the testimonies come from people I know, such as those on my personal team who pray for all my books as they are being written (and pray for you as you are reading them). Other testimonies come from people I have never met but who have read some of my previous books and have answered yes to my social media appeal to participate. These people all have one thing in common: They did what you are about to do and were healed.

By the way, in case you are new to using essential oils and are not quite sure what to do with the "Apply" section of my A-lists in these next chapters, let me fill you in. You can use the A-list oils either one at a time or by mixing them together as a blend in a "carrier oil," as I am about to describe just ahead. (Please note that a blend is always going to be more powerful.) Once you choose the oil (or oils) you will use, there are three ways you can get them into your system:

1. *You can apply the oils directly on the body.*

    Orally: You can take some essential oils by mouth, either via a few drops in a capsule, or in a water tonic (5 drops maximum). Check the bottle to see if the oil you have is safe to ingest.

    Topically: Apply the oil directly on your skin. Either apply a maximum of 5 drops "neat" (directly on the skin, without dilution), or apply a maximum of 5 drops per teaspoon of carrier oil (the carrier can be olive oil, grape seed, almond, sesame, fractionated coconut, etc.). Look online or on the back of your essential oil bottle to see if it can be applied neat or not. You can apply the drops to your pulse points (wrists), temples, neck, brain stem region (the back of your neck, just under the hairline), the bottoms of your feet, or directly on the region of discomfort (but never in your eyes).

2. *You can use essential oils in the air.* Essential oils are helpful and healthful when used in general

aromatherapy. Try the following to help you breathe more deeply or liven up any living space:

Apply 2 drops on a tissue or handkerchief and place it over your nose (or under your pillowcase at night) for deep breathing. Or hold the bottle under your nose and breathe deeply. The oil goes directly to the limbic areas of your brain through the nasal passages for rapid effect.

Utilize the following aromatherapy tools to enjoy the scent of the oils in the air:

 » Diffusers that activate the oil and release it into the air—use 1–6 drops.
 » Lightbulbs—apply 1 drop on a cool bulb, and it will smell once the bulb is switched on.
 » Fireplace wood—apply 3 drops per log, using pine, cypress or cedarwood oil.
 » Candles—use 2 drops in a candle once lit and heated, avoiding the wick.
 » Humidifiers—use 2–8 drops directly in the water; refill and repeat.
 » Spray bottles—use 5 drops in warm water in bottle, then shake.

3. *You can use essential oils in water.* We all know our skin has a million little mouths on it, which is why what you soak in seeps in.
 • Bath—Add 8–10 drops after the water is drawn; soak and breathe.
 • Epsom salt bath—Add 10 drops per cup of salts in warm water.
 • Shower—Add 2 drops on your scalp or 4 drops on a cloth to scrub your skin.

- Footbath—Add 4–6 drops in warm water; soak for 15 minutes.
- Spot bath—Add 3 drops in water; soak any area (hands, etc.).

Also take note of a few special considerations when using essential oils on your children or pets. When applying essential oils to small children, use a carrier oil. Consult your pediatrician first if you feel the oils may interfere with any medical regimens already prescribed for your kids. Always research your essential oils online before applying them to your pets. In some articles, pet owners have reported adverse affects with oil application or contact, while I have others who say that they have applied my Quiet Brain essential oil blend to their pets with great and relaxing results. Proper research and reaching out to your veterinarian will help you find answers to any questions you may have about pet safety and essential oils.

Testimony

"Reading through the declarations and blessings has brought me to the realization that I have allowed myself to hold on to sickness for far too long. I have said no to opportunities, events and even jobs based on the chaos that was happening in my body, fearful that I would not be able to perform my best due to what was happening in that moment rather than (1) taking hold of my healing and taking a step of faith, (2) saying yes to all He has for me and (3) truly accepting I was healed that very moment and not allowing sickness to rob me of a healthy future. I'm happy to say that after reading these body system blessings, I have now fearlessly stepped into my divine purpose and am fiercely maintaining my miracle!" ~Bryant

11

Nervous System

Brain, Spinal Cord, Nerves

Declaration

I am ready to receive any needed healing for my nervous system and then do whatever it takes to walk in divine health. I know that God does not make me sick, and I ask Him right now to show me the root of my condition, whether it be physical, emotional or spiritual. I am ready to pray the prayer of faith, reverse the curse and unleash the blessing. By God's grace, I will watch my words, maintain my miracle or wait on God's perfect timing for healing. Amen!

Nervous System Blessing

Your central nervous system—comprised of your brain and spinal cord—are healthy and at peace. Your peripheral nervous system—the nerve fibers that branch off from the spinal cord and extend to every part of

Nervous System

your body, including each organ—communicates perfectly with your whole body and mind. Your more than 100 billion neurons fire perfectly and are adequately coated in myelin, and you have optimum function in each axon, dendrite, neurotransmitter, nucleus and synapse. Your cerebrum and its left and right hemispheres, and the corpus callosum that connects them, are sound. Each hemisphere's lobe—frontal, temporal, parietal and occipital—results in healthy white matter and gray matter, and your thalamus and hypothalamus control each part of your body and your hormone production with perfection. Your mental health is also perfect, with your body free from all chemical imbalances that would affect your moods. Your spinal cord, brain stem and cerebrospinal fluid are conduits of health to your whole body. The leptomeninges and dura mater are now providing a healthy protective shield to guard every blessing your nervous system has just received. Let it be done according to your faith and in the mighty name of Jesus!

Visit lauraharrissmith.com/blessings for the video blessing.

Your Nervous System's A-list

Avoid caffeine, sugar, wheat, dairy, alcohol, commercial fruit juices, aspartame, MSG

Add avocados, almond flour, leafy greens, steroid-free organic meats; herbs: chamomile, valerian, lemon balm, skullcap and other nervines; *rest*

Allow fish oil; magnesium taurate; vitamins B complex, D3, E; flax and chia seeds

Apply Quiet Brain, frankincense, lavender, cedarwood, sandalwood oils

Anoint with oil daily and pray necessary healing prayers and body system blessings

Ask your doctor or health care professional before making regimen changes

Your Nervous System's Favorite . . .

Breakfast: steel-cut oatmeal with stevia or Swerve and cinnamon; egg/spinach/veggie omelet

Lunch: leafy green salad with almonds, avocado, tomato; organic chicken

Dinner: broccoli with garlic in olive oil; spinach salad with quinoa; fatty fish or organic chicken

Snack: 70–80 percent cocoa organic dark chocolate (I recommend Lily's brand, made with stevia), nuts, pumpkin seeds, hummus, cucumbers

Testimony

"My Grandma Arlene had a seizure and no one was with her. My parents found her unresponsive. Mom quickly got Laura's Quiet Brain oil. I also prayed the nervous system blessing over her. Most of the time she would have had to go to the ER and be hospitalized, but in just a couple of hours she was talking to us and doing her normal activities. It would have normally taken her days. A few days ago, she started shaking and Mom ran into the other room and put the Quiet Brain on her, and she felt more relaxed. All the shaking stopped entirely (without a seizure ever starting). She hadn't had any episodes in a very long time, so this was the first time we got to try Quiet Brain on her and pray the nervous system body blessing over her. She is doing amazingly well." ~Jennifer

> After reading the blessings and prayers, send all testimonies large and small to healing@lauraharrissmith.com.

Nervous System Healing Prayers

Alzheimer's Disease Healing Prayer

God, we speak calm and courage over the frightening diagnosis of Alzheimer's. Let the faith in my heart bring healing to my brain. I declare that my 100 billion brain cells are free of plaques—deposits of the protein beta-amyloid trying to build up in between my nerve cells. And my brain is free of all tangles—the twisted fibers of the protein tau trying to build up inside my brain cells. I believe, O God, that You do not want me confused, because 1 Corinthians 14:33 says, "For God is not a God of confusion but of peace." I speak directly to the mood changes, disorientation and the suspicions about my family, friends and caregivers, and I speak a blessing over those caregivers for serving me. Physically, I thank You that I will not have difficulty speaking, remembering, swallowing, walking or anything else I want to do, as soon as I want to do it! Holy Spirit, come. Rejuvenate my memory and the hippocampus of my brain to accomplish this. Bless any medications or nutritional supplements I am on, and protect me from side effects. I declare that Alzheimer's is just a name and that Jesus has the name above all names. In His name I pray, Amen.

Amyotrophic Lateral Sclerosis (ALS / Lou Gehrig's Disease) Healing Prayer

Jesus, this diagnosis and the prognosis that comes with it are intimidating, but You are my Healer, so I am unafraid of the future. I declare that I will live out all the days You have for me on this earth, and I claim Psalm 118:17 for my very own: "I shall not die, but I shall live, and recount the deeds of the Lord." Father, please protect the motor neurons in my brain so that this disease cannot kill them and prevent me from walking, talking, grasping, eating, moving, breathing and anything else I need to do to live, love, work and enjoy my life. I speak life over my brain, spinal cord and entire nervous system, and declare that I will progressively get stronger, not weaker. I speak life into my muscular system and declare that my muscles will be nourished and not atrophy. Holy Spirit, come. Bless any medications or nutritional supplements I am on, and protect me from side effects, God. I also trust You to protect my family from any genetic inheritance of this disease. As You heal me, You are healing them. In Jesus' name, Amen.

Autism Healing Prayer

Lord, first we deal with the disappointment of this diagnosis and cast our cares entirely upon You as Healer. In the mighty name of Jesus, we bind the deaf and dumb spirit You mention in Mark 9, since autism is also a disorder that causes a disruption in listening, hearing and general communication and social skills. We speak to _____'s brain and command it to be healed in the tiny, unknown crevices in which doctors do not even understand why or how they were afflicted. You are the Great Physician, Jesus. We declare that all tormenting repetitive motions will cease, and that calm will settle in during moments of potential outbursts and anger. Father, if You choose a progressive healing instead of an instant miracle, then show us the right people to teach us and the right homeopathic remedies to cure this. Modern medicine currently has none, but homeopathic (not just naturopathic) remedies have done wonders in rescuing many children out of autism's grasp. Holy Spirit, come. We await Your guidance. In Jesus' name, Amen.

Brain Damage Healing Prayer

In the mighty name of Jesus we reverse the curse of brain damage. Whatever the cause, whatever the injury, whatever the prognosis, we declare that the mind of _____ is whole and restored. We bind the Mark 9 deaf and dumb spirit in the name of Jesus, and we ask God to make it as if this craniocerebral trauma never happened. Please heal all blurred vision, confusion, difficulty concentrating and learning, immobility, amnesia, inability to create new memories, abnormal outbursts of crying or laughing, irritability, aggression, lack of restraint, incontinence, nausea, unequal pupils, headache, seizures and loneliness. Healing, come! Speech, come! Damaged cells, go! I pray for perfect rest at night and during the day, and that you would guide the medical professionals working with us with the wisdom of Solomon. Bless any medications or nutritional supplements You guide us by Your Spirit to use. Holy Spirit, come. We pray now and release the mind of Christ over this situation, and believe that this person will be "transformed by the renewal" of the mind (Romans 12:2). In Your name, Lord, Amen.

Cerebral Palsy Healing Prayer

Father, right now we need You to rewrite the broken DNA in _____'s brain. Whether the palsy came from genetic mutation, maternal infection, fetal stroke, a head injury, a complicated birth or a premature, undeveloped brain, it matters not, because You can override them all. We ask for help with speaking, hearing, eating, sucking, touching, walking, bladder control and more. Heal any muscle imbalance in the eyes so that this person can see more clearly, heal all brain waves so that they can fire more calmly and heal all spasticity, ataxia and athetosis so that every muscle functions as You intended. May not a single muscle shorten or become rigid, thanks to Your merciful might, and we declare that whatever has already shortened or atrophied will begin to regrow. We assert by Christ's authority that a perfect relationship between nervous system and muscular system exists in this body. We also proclaim that intellect will be released and communication will increase, and Father, even quicken the imagination to come alive and to begin creating. Holy Spirit, come. We say in faith "be renewed in the spirit of your mind" (Ephesians

4:23 NASB). We also thank You for the grace that has rested upon us up until now to walk this hard road, but we believe You for a different road . . . an easier road . . . and for strong, healed legs to travel to new places and proclaim what You have done for us. In Jesus' name, Amen.

Concussion (Mild Traumatic Brain Injury) Healing Prayer

Lord, thank You for being my Protector during this injury that could have been so much worse. But now, I turn to You as Healer from all these temporary cognitive symptoms. Please bring remedy and relief to the lack of coordination, abnormal fatigue, depression, memory loss, nausea, ringing in the ears, confusion and headache. Jesus, please reduce the swelling from impact and stabilize my brain waves as my neurons are communicating better to one another daily. Please resolve all light and sound sensitivities and bring peace to my entire nervous system. Holy Spirit, come. I ask You to return me quickly to my original state of mind, and even better! Guard my sleep from any disturbances and help me rest as You bring about perfect health for me. Finally, give grace to those around me whom this injury is impacting, whether they be family, friends or co-workers, for I value their patience and ask You to reward it. "And we know that for those who love God all things work together for good, for those who are called according to his purpose" (Romans 8:28). In Your name, Amen.

Dementia (Memory Loss) Healing Prayer

Lord, Proverbs 10:7 tells me, "The memory of the righteous is blessed" (NKJV), so I ask You to guard every memory I have from the life You have given me on earth, and do not let a single one be stolen from me. Holy Spirit, come. Help me focus. Help me remember. Help me continue doing the tasks I have to do to care for myself, but I thank You for those people whom You have brought to help care for me. Bless any medications or nutritional supplements I am on, and protect me from side effects. I declare that my brain cells will communicate perfectly with one another, in the name of Jesus. I thank You that as I work to memorize Scripture, You are going to quicken my brain to heal and retain, and I declare that the hippocampus of my brain is going to grow progressively better, not progressively worse. I am not afraid of the future, because I know You are already there. I pray this in the name of Jesus, Amen.

Epilepsy (Seizures) Healing Prayer

It is in the mighty name of Jesus that we serve notice to the Mark 9 deaf and dumb spirit, the only spirit in Scripture that Jesus gave a name to, doing so as He delivered the little epileptic boy from its merciless grasp. We declare to it that this same exact deliverance is ours today, so we pray the prayer in Mark 9:24: "I do believe; help my unbelief" (NASB). I speak peace—shalom—right now over my brain (or _____'s brain) and command the neurons to fire properly and communicate with each other without interruption or overactivity. We renounce the thievery of time and consciousness and declare that every moment stolen will be returned tenfold, with longer life. We release healing and relief from all forms of seizures—grand mal convulsions, petit mal "absence" seizures, tonic-clonic, myoclonic, atonic—and regardless of whether they are idiopathic, cryptogenic, symptomatic, generalized, focal or partial, we command them to go in the name of Jesus. Father, return joy for every moment spent in anxiety, depression and fear. We speak a blessing in place of every headache, paralysis and bruise suffered. We also speak blessing to our caretakers, knowing that it is often harder on those who watch. Holy Spirit, come. Remind me to adhere to this chapter's A-list for optimum neurological health. Thank You for total healing, O great God! In Your name, Lord, Amen.

Fainting (Syncope) Healing Prayer

Jesus, strengthen me and bring to light the reasons why I am losing consciousness. Mend the relationship between my circulatory system and nervous system so that I might have ample blood supply to my brain and never lose consciousness again (syncope). Holy Spirit, come. Please regulate my heart rate and blood pressure, and instruct my vagus nerve to do its job with perfection. I trust You with my very life, Lord, and will not be afraid. I proclaim this promise over myself: "You brought up my life from the pit, O LORD my God. When my life was fainting away, I remembered the LORD, and my prayer came to you, into your holy temple" (Jonah 2:6–7). In Jesus' name I pray, Amen.

Huntington's Disease Healing Prayer

Jesus, my future is in Your hands, and I have no reason to be afraid, despite this intimidating diagnosis. I declare, in Your mighty name, that my nervous system is strong and that my nerve cells are growing stronger over time and not weaker. They will not break down, and I will not become a statistic. Proverbs 18:21 tells me that the power of life and death is in my tongue, so I speak life, life, life to my entire body and my ability to walk, speak and concentrate. Holy Spirit, come. I have faith that You can protect me from devastating symptoms like memory loss, involuntary movements, coordination issues, muscle loss and spasms, confusion, delusion, difficulty reasoning, or lack of restraint, and I also ask You to remove this illness from my family line and let it stop with me. I declare over my mind that I will be full of joy. I will not be depressed, anxious, apathetic or angry. And I will not have my voice stolen. As long as there is breath in my lungs, I will praise Jehovah Rapha, my Healer. "So I will bless you as long as I live; in Your name I will lift up my hands. My soul will be satisfied as with fat and rich food, and my mouth will praise you with joyful lips. When I remember you upon my bed, and meditate on you in the watches of the night; for you have been my help, and in the shadow of your wings I will sing for joy. My soul clings to you; your right hand upholds me" (Psalm 63:4–8). In Jesus' name, Amen.

Meningitis Healing Prayer

Lord, my body wants to be racked with pain, but my heart wants to trust You. The spirit is willing, but the flesh is weak, so I put my spirit in the driver's seat right now and declare that You are in control. I speak healing over the membranes that surround my brain—the meninges—and I command the inflammation and swelling to leave them. I also rebuke the debilitating headache, fever and stiff neck. Holy Spirit, come. Deliver me from chronic pain! And by God's authority I say, "Spirit of pain, leave!" Whether this affliction is viral, bacterial or fungal, I resist it, and I thank You, God, that You are improving my overall health every day. I receive peace instead of irritability, hunger instead of appetite loss, clear skin instead of rashes, clarity instead of confusion, alertness instead of grogginess and joy instead of sorrow. Isaiah 53:4–5 says, "Surely he has borne our griefs and carried our sorrows; yet we esteemed him stricken, smitten by God, and afflicted. But he was pierced for our transgressions; he was crushed for our iniquities; upon him was the chastisement that brought us peace, and with his wounds we are healed." And I believe it. In Jesus' name, Amen.

Migraine Healing Prayer

Father, in the name of Your Son I cry out to You for healing from these migraine headaches. I am weary of the throbbing, the isolation and the agonizing pain. I speak to this condition—which neurologists call a "slow motion seizure"—and in Your name I command it to go. I also resist the intense nausea, sensitivity to light, vision loss and inability to speak clearly. God, whether it is in the prodromal stage in the days before (which includes the mood swings, yawning and neck stiffness) or the aura stage (during which I experience the speech and vision changes), I declare that I will call upon Your name and You will deliver me from this enemy. I believe that You can and want to prevent me from ever living through another attack phase and the postdrome phase that follows, with all its vomiting, headache hangover and more. Holy Spirit, come. Remind me to adhere to this chapter's A-list for optimum neurological health. You are my peace, God, and "You keep him in perfect peace whose mind is stayed on you, because he trusts in you" (Isaiah 26:3). And I do. In Your name, Amen.

Neuropathy Healing Prayer

In the name of Jesus I command this peripheral neuropathy to leave my body. You are not welcome in my hands, in my feet, my back, face or thighs. Father, I ask You to recreate the nerves in those places and restore them to perfect condition. Deliver me from the intense burning and tingling in my extremities, God, not to mention the loss of muscle and lack of coordination. Remove the cramping and help me regain my footing and balance. "You have not delivered me into the hand of the enemy; you have set my feet in a broad place," says the psalmist (Psalm 31:8), and I claim the same blessing for myself. Holy Spirit, come. Help me sleep in peace at night and be pain free during the day. God, show me if diet is playing a part in this, and teach me Your nutritional wisdom so that I might walk in divine health. I do not want to be on medications and ointments that treat pain but not the underlying condition, so show me the root of this illness and I will cooperate with You to usher in healing. Thank You, Lord! In Your name, Amen.

Paralysis Healing Prayer

God, my brain has not been communicating well with my muscles. I know You see exactly where the breakdown is, and You can see what the medical tests cannot and bring healing where the doctors are left scratching their heads. I thank You for Your grace to live my life as I am, but I do not believe it is Your best for me to live as a paraplegic, quadriplegic or with any paralysis at all in my body or face, so I will resist all of the above in prayer. Jesus, touch my nervous, skeletal and muscular systems and cause my nerves, bones and muscles to work together to produce vitality and mobility in my body. Holy Spirit, come. I will be at peace and declare Psalm 116:7–9 over myself: "Return, O my soul, to your rest; for the LORD has dealt bountifully with you. For you have delivered my soul from death, my eyes from tears, my feet from stumbling; I will walk before the LORD in the land of the living." I believe it! Your will be done in my body, O God. In the name of Jesus, Amen.

Parkinson's Disease Healing Prayer

God, I refuse to be discouraged or afraid at the diagnosis of Parkinson's. It is just a name, and You have the name above all names, Jesus. So, while the facts tell me that my body is shaking with tremors and that my brain is ailing, the truth is that I am healed by You. I declare right now that the facts will submit themselves to the truth, and that I will be Parkinson's free. I command my brain to be well and to make all the dopamine my neurons need in the substantia nigra, which is the nucleus in my midbrain that controls my movements. I refuse the nonmotor symptoms of insomnia, constipation, depression and the loss of a sense of smell, as well as the motor symptoms, which affect my movements. I will be coordinated. I will keep my balance. I will not fall, and I will not tremble. I command my body to receive the healing God has for me, and I command my mind and emotions to be content as God rewires my nervous, muscular and sensory systems altogether. I speak over my body Hebrews 12:12–13: "Therefore, strengthen the hands that are weak and the knees that are feeble, and make straight paths for your feet, so that the limb which is lame may not be put out of joint, but rather be healed" (NASB). Holy Spirit, come. In Jesus' name, Amen.

Pinched Nerves Healing Prayer

God, my body is in great need of a touch from You. It cries out in pain day and night for relief. I ask You to relieve the pressure that my nerves are receiving from their surrounding bones, muscles, cartilage, tendons and any other tissue. Give me a holy realignment and cause my skeletal system and muscular system to be good to my nervous system and not invade the spaces You have given it to occupy. I speak life to my limbs and body, and I rebuke the numbness, burning, pain, pins-and-needles tingling, and the constant sensation of my limbs falling asleep. God, please give me better sleep at night—peaceful sleep—and I declare what Psalm 127:2 says about You over myself: "He gives His beloved sleep" (NKJV). Whatever is causing the compression to my nerves, O God , mend it, whether it be from stress, arthritis or an injury. And God, if this is something that I can alleviate myself by losing weight, then I vow to You that with Your help, I will make the necessary changes to eat healthier and lose weight. Holy Spirit, come. Thank You for healing and grace. I pray this in Your name, Amen.

Sciatica Healing Prayer

In addition to the healing prayer that I prayed (or will pray) about pinched nerves, I say by faith that I also know You are healing my sciatic nerve that has been causing this pain, which seems to afflict various areas stretching from my back down to my calf. I declare I will be pain free and suffer no more from the accompanying weakness and the bladder or bowel changes. Holy Spirit, come. I speak Isaiah 43:2 over the burning in my legs and body: "When you walk through fire you shall not be burned, and the flame shall not consume you." I trust You for healing, God. In Jesus' name, Amen.

Spinal Cord Injury Healing Prayer

O great and merciful God, my future is in Your hands. From the moment of my injury, everything beneath the break—or the impact my spinal cord sustained—seemed to die, along with all the movement I enjoyed, which was controlled by that area. You were there. You kept me alive. You have a purpose for me that I am determined to fulfill, sitting or standing. But since James 4:2 says "Ye have not, because ye ask not" (KJV), it will not be said of me that I do not ask You for healing. So Lord, I ask You right now to recreate what died beneath that point of impact on my spinal cord. Rejuvenate the nerves, bones, cartilage and tendons so that I might feel, walk, run, dance, have bowel and bladder control and be independent again. I welcome the sensation back into my limbs and body! I declare that my nervous, skeletal and muscular systems will work together in harmony. I command my muscles not to atrophy, my nerves to be calm and the painful muscle spasms and overactive reflexes to cease. I surrender to You my feelings of abandonment, embarrassment, depression and anger, and I speak a blessing over my caretakers, who have not given up on me. Should You choose a progressive healing for me, Lord, give us wisdom about health professionals, medications, supplements and therapy. Holy Spirit, come. By faith, I see myself whole and proclaim that "I will walk before the LORD in the land of the living" (Psalm 116:9). In Jesus' name, Amen.

TIA (Transient Ischemic Attack; Mini-Stroke) Healing Prayer

Jesus, this experience has been difficult, but I know that the battle belongs to You and not to me. I know that You alone can heal this muscle weakness, numbness, light-headedness, vertigo, confusion, slurred speech and blurred vision. I know that You can return to me my coordination, mobility and the ability to eat, drink, walk, run and even dance if I want to. So I am asking You to do all of the above. Holy Spirit, come. Be glorified through my healing, and restore to me the youthfulness that only You can recreate. Finally, I declare that this episode will not be a precursor to another stroke, for my nervous system is being healed even as we speak, and the healing is spreading to my muscular and sensory systems, as well. I declare over myself—body, mind and spirit— Joel 3:10: "Let the weak say, I am strong" (KJV). In the name of Jesus, Amen.

Tremor (Essential Tremor) Healing Prayer

Lord, when I feel out of control or afraid, I know You are with me always, because You tell me so in Matthew 28:20 and I believe in Your Word. But You also tell me in Exodus 15:26 that You are my Healer, so I am coming to You today for just that— healing. God, You know the exact source of this tremor, and I am asking You to touch it right now and bring peace to it. Holy Spirit, come. Cause my nervous system to work correctly with my endocrine and muscular systems to bring calm to my entire body. Bless my hands as I hold them out to You right now, Lord, and grant them strength and healing so that they might write, type, eat, shave and do so many other necessary things, including completing the work You have given me to do on this earth. Help me stay rested and free of constant stress, so that my body does not respond negatively. I claim this verse as my own, God: "'Though the mountains be shaken and the hills be removed, yet my unfailing love for you will not be shaken nor my covenant of peace be removed,' says the LORD, who has compassion on you" (Isaiah 54:10 NIV). In Jesus' name, Amen.

12

Sensory System

Sight, Hearing, Feeling, Smelling, Tasting, Balance

Declaration

I am ready to receive any needed healing for my sensory system and then do whatever it takes to walk in divine health. I know that God does not make me sick, and I ask Him right now to show me the root of my condition, whether it be physical, emotional or spiritual. I am ready to pray the prayer of faith, reverse the curse and unleash the blessing. By God's grace, I will watch my words, maintain my miracle or wait on God's perfect timing for healing. Amen!

Sensory System Blessing

All five of your sensory system's sense organs—your eyes, ears, tongue, nose and skin—are being restored

Sensory System

right now back to their youthful conditions. Your chemoreceptors (on skin, mouth and nose) and your photoreceptors (eyes) and mechanoreceptors (ears) are all attentive and healthy. Your taste buds, microvilli, nasal cavity, sinuses and brain all have the proper nerve impulses necessary for you to enjoy the healthy foods God has provided for you to eat. Your eardrums' tiny bones—the malleus, incus and stapes—work perfectly in conjunction with the inner ears' hair cells, cilia, semicircular canals and vestibule to provide you with perfect hearing, balance and equilibrium. Your eyes are blessed with sharpness and youthfulness in your pupils, corneas, lenses, ciliary muscles, optic nerves, vitreous bodies, retinas and photoreceptors. Let it be done according to your faith and in the mighty name of Jesus!

Visit lauraharrissmith.com/blessings for the video blessing.

Your Sensory System's A-list

Avoid caffeine, dairy, sugar, cakes, fried foods, alcohol, soda, red meat

Add walnuts, carrots, avocados, leafy greens, fish, eggs, organic poultry

Allow vitamins A, B complex, C; apple cider vinegar (ACV), zinc, fish oil, flax and chia seeds, lutein

Apply lemon, peppermint or lavender oil in cupped hands over nose; diffuse

Anoint with oil daily and pray needed healing prayers and body system blessings

Ask your doctor or health care provider before making regimen changes

Your Sensory System's Favorite . . .

Breakfast: egg and veggie omelet with turmeric; fresh green juice; citrus (grapefruit)

Lunch: sweet potato with coconut oil, grated ginger and cinnamon; sautéed carrots with olive oil

Dinner: green veggie salad with walnuts, tomato, olive oil, lemon; organic chicken with fresh dill

Snack: sunflower seeds, cashews, citrus, melon, carrots, red pepper, avocado with cayenne pepper; water

Testimony

"I felt a cold coming on with a sore throat and read Laura's sensory system blessing for my ears, nose, throat, eyes, sinuses, etc. I also combined some of the foods from the list for a soothing drink: 1 cup hot water with 1 tablespoon ACV, 1 tablespoon lemon juice, 1 tablespoon honey (I normally don't use honey due to the glycemic spike, but it really coats the throat when sore) and 1 teaspoon cinnamon. Between both natural *and* supernatural remedies, my sore throat was literally gone the next day, and the cold never came on!" ~Lee

After reading the blessings and prayers, send all testimonies large and small to healing@lauraharrissmith.com.

Sensory System Healing Prayers

Common Cold Healing Prayer

God, I cannot afford to be out for a week or two with a cold, so I am asking You to reverse the virus I've come in contact with and remove it from my body. Take with it the runny nose, drainage, congestion, sore throat, sneezing, sinus pressure, phlegm and fatigue. On the other hand, Lord, I hear experts saying that we do not catch a cold; we earn it. In other words, many say there is no cure for the common cold because it is less of an illness and more of a detox after not taking care of yourself, with mucus being the mechanism You created for toxins to jump into and exit the body (while coughing or blowing a congested nose). In light of that, I ask Your forgiveness for consuming too much of the wrong foods and getting too little of the right kind of deep sleep that my immune system needs to ward off illness. I praise you for the miracle of a fever, which is evidence that my immune system is working hard to fight for my recovery. Holy Spirit, come. I pray for total cleansing and healing to my body, and I thank You, God, that I am "fearfully and wonderfully made" (Psalm 139:14). In the name of Jesus, Amen.

Conjunctivitis (Pink Eye) Healing Prayer

In the name of Jesus I command this contagious infection to go. The inflammation and irritation in my eyes is being healed even now. O Lord, whether it is viral or bacterial, please take away the infection and its pain, discharge, puffiness, redness, swelling and sensitivity to light. I declare that my circulatory system and sensory system will work together so that there is adequate blood flow into my eyes to expedite healing in the tiny blood vessels of the conjunctiva. Holy Spirit, come. I claim Matthew 9:29 for my own: "Then He touched their eyes, saying, 'It shall be done to you according to your faith'" (NASB). In Jesus' name, Amen.

147

Ear Infection (Acute Otitis Media) Healing Prayer

Lord, thank You for my immune system, which You have designed to resist the infection trying to overtake my sensory system—specifically, my ears. Holy Spirit, come. I turn to You for healing from the ear pain, drainage, headache, loss of balance and impaired hearing, and I declare that I will be able to lie down in peace without worsening pain. I praise You for the miracle of a fever, God, which is evidence that my immune system is working hard to fight for my recovery. I declare victory to it, as You intend. "He who has ears to hear, let him hear" (Matthew 11:15). In Jesus' name, Amen.

Eye Conditions (Including Blindness) Healing Prayer

Lord, I know You want my eyes to see clearly so that I might serve You without hindrance, so I am asking You to heal and protect them from any and all of the following: blindness, nearsightedness, farsightedness, chronic dry eye, glaucoma, cataracts, age-related macular degeneration, lazy eye, corneal abrasion, corneal ulcer, retinal detachment or tearing, astigmatisms, presbyopia, amblyopia, ocular hypertension, uveitis, strabismus (crossed eyes), bulging eyes, blocked tear ducts, dacrocystitis, blepharitis, diabetic retinopathy, diabetic macular edema, keratoconus, CMV retinitis, eye flashes, anisocoria, double vision (diplopia), eye strokes, Fuchs' corneal dystrophy, hyphema, nystagmus, milia, optic neuropathy, peripheral vision loss, photophobia, eyelid twitches and yes, even color blindness. Holy Spirit, come. Heal every part of my eyes by Your power and in Your timing. "Moved with compassion, Jesus touched their eyes; and immediately they regained their sight and followed Him" (Matthew 20:34 NASB). I thank You in advance for healed eyes, Lord. In Your name, Amen.

Hearing Loss (Including Deafness) Healing Prayer

Jehovah Rapha, I am asking You to heal these ears so that they might hear all the beautiful sounds in Your world. The sounds of creation, the sounds of loved ones and even the sounds that keep me safe and able to live and drive independently. Please cause my nervous and sensory systems to work perfectly in harmony, so that any nerve damage can be reversed and I can hear with total clarity. Heal my eardrums' tiny bones—the malleus, incus and stapes—and cause them to work perfectly in conjunction with my inner ears' hair cells, cilia, semicircular canals and vestibule, providing me with perfect hearing and equilibrium. Provide healing for both conductive hearing loss and sensorineural hearing loss. Holy Spirit, come. Luke 22:51 says, "But Jesus answered and said, 'Stop! No more of this.' And He touched his ear and healed him" (NASB). I receive that today in Jesus' name, Amen.

Laryngitis Healing Prayer

Lord, I may not be able to pray this in full voice, but I believe that if I begin to try, You will heal me as I speak by faith, and You will continue to heal me all day. I pray You would heal the inflammation in my vocal cords and swelling in my larynx, regardless of its origin. Remove any accompanying cough, sore throat, frequent clearing, congestion, runny nose, phlegm and fatigue. Holy Spirit, come. I receive Your invitation to make the changes necessary for better health, adhering to this chapter's A-list nutritional advice. Help me rest well and use this opportunity to listen better . . . to You and to others. I declare Psalm 71:8 over myself: "My mouth is filled with your praise, declaring your splendor all day long" (NLT). In Jesus' name, Amen.

Ménière's Disease Healing Prayer

Lord, please touch my inner ear and specifically my vestibular system, which provides me with my balance. Decrease the swelling inside my cochlea and reduce the water retention involved in this condition. Holy Spirit, come. Please deliver me from the ringing and buzzing (tinnitus), nausea, dizziness, ear pain, uncontrolled eye movements, diarrhea, fatigue, mood changes, cold sweats, constant pressure, migraines and lack of balance and coordination. "He will not let your foot slip" (Psalm 121:3 NIV). I trust You to answer my prayer and restore my sensory system and ears in Jesus' name. Amen.

Nosebleeds Healing Prayer

Note: As a very little girl, my first encounter with the Word of God healing me was with a dangerous nosebleed while visiting my grandmother's house ten hours away from my parents. When none of Granny's remedies stopped the hour-long nosebleed, she called church friend after church friend in her tiny town, trying to remember "the Bible verse that would heal nosebleeds." I had never heard of such a thing, nor had I experienced God's Word being used in this way. Finally, a neighbor told her the verse, and as she read it over me, the bleeding stopped. The fear of the Lord came upon me, and I will never forget the miracle. Now I share this verse with you today, especially since it is good not only for nosebleeds, but for so much more! Rather than a long prayer here, just speak Isaiah 53:5 (NKJV) over yourself, as Granny did over me:

"But He was wounded for our transgressions, He was bruised for our iniquities; the chastisement for our peace was upon Him, and by His stripes we are healed." Holy Spirit, come. In the name of Jesus, who has purchased every healing I will ever need, I command this nosebleed to stop and be healed, along with any underlying condition causing it. In His name, Amen.

Ringing in Ears (Tinnitus) Healing Prayer

In the name of Jesus, I command this ringing in my ears to cease! Also, the roaring, hissing, buzzing and all other annoying sounds. Whether it is subjective tinnitus (where only I can hear the sounds) or objective tinnitus (where even others can hear them, too), I ask for peace in my ears and head, in Jesus' name. Mend any ear damage I have incurred, whether it came through exposure to loud sounds or from medications. But Lord, if the ringing is a symptom of something more dangerous, then I ask You to help us discover and cure whatever that is. Holy Spirit, come. Heal me from any high blood pressure, high cholesterol, TMJ and middle-ear muscle spasms, and show me how to walk in divine health and take better care of myself so that my ears might find peace. I ask all of this, Lord, knowing that You say, "Take care then how you hear" (Luke 8:18). In Your name I pray, Amen.

Sinusitis (Sinus Infection) Healing Prayer

Jesus, laying my own hands on my face, skull, ears and head as I pray, I ask You to relieve me of this sinus pain and swelling in my sinus cavities, now. Whether triggered by allergies or a cold, I declare that this will not become a chronic condition and last the typical eight to twelve weeks. In fact, I believe that You are resolving this infirmity even as I pray, and healing any nasal polyps or even a deviated septum, if that is to blame. I rebuke the congestion, tenderness, headache, breathing difficulties, sleeplessness, throat irritation, runny nose, loss of smell, and fatigue, and I release by faith in You Your healing power into my body, clearing both my head and mind. Holy Spirit, come. I receive Genesis 2:7: "Then the LORD God formed the man of dust from the ground and breathed into his nostrils the breath of life, and the man became a living creature." In Your name, Jesus, Amen.

Strep Throat Healing Prayer

God, I ask You please to bring me relief. I need healing from this group A streptococcus bacteria in my body. Holy Spirit, come. I ask You to remove the sore throat, chills, swollen tonsils, headache, fatigue, and the nausea and misery. Lord, let my immune system battle for healing even if a fever arises, which would be a good sign that it is strong and fighting, and I receive Your invitation to make the changes necessary for better health, adhering to this chapter's A-list nutritional advice. I command the infection in my body to surrender to God's healing power right now, and for the swollen lymph glands to properly drain the infection and quickly return to their normal, pain-free size. "I am weary of my crying: my throat is dried: mine eyes fail while I wait for my God" (Psalm 69:3 KJV). I ask all this in Your miracle-working name, Amen.

Vertigo Healing Prayer

Psalm 119:173 says, "Put your hand out and steady me" (MESSAGE), and that is exactly what I need You to do, Lord. Holy Spirit, come. Heal me of the sensations of spinning, tilting, swaying, falling and dizziness, and the resulting symptoms of nausea, headache and fatigue. Dissolve any calcium particles (canaliths) in my inner ear canals that might be causing benign paroxysmal positional vertigo (BPPV). Jesus, if there has been any labyrinthitis due to a viral infection, please reduce the inflammation in my inner ear and mend the surrounding nerves. Show me, or those caring for me, if the vertigo is a symptom of a greater problem, whether it be neurological or skeletal, and then extend Your healing hand to that issue, as well. I ask all this in Your powerful name, Amen.

13

Endocrine System

Hypothalamus, Pituitary, Thyroid, Adrenals, Pineal Body

Declaration

I am ready to receive any needed healing for my endocrine system and then do whatever it takes to walk in divine health. I know that God does not make me sick, and I ask Him right now to show me the root of my condition, whether it be physical, emotional or spiritual. I am ready to pray the prayer of faith, reverse the curse and unleash the blessing. By God's grace, I will watch my words, maintain my miracle or wait on God's perfect timing for healing. Amen!

Endocrine System Blessing

I release a blessing of health upon your endocrine system and the many glands that comprise it. Your

Endocrine System

hypothalamus adequately connects your nervous system to your endocrine system and fulfills its main job of telling your pituitary gland (the body's master gland) to make or stop making all of your body's hormones. Your pituitary adapts promptly to what the body needs and to what the hypothalamus commands, and you are thereby able to manage stress, blood sugar and weight, and even bring forth children, if desired. Your pineal gland makes the necessary melatonin for you to sleep well, and your thyroid is "rebooting" right now to regulate your metabolism, weight, heart rate, body temperature and energy. I speak divine health over your parathyroid for bone health, your thymus to fight infection, your pancreas to break down food and regulate insulin, and your adrenals so that you can make adrenaline and cortisol and have boundless energy and manage stress. Finally, I release a blessing over your reproductive hormones that will see you through all the phases of your life with graceful transitions. Let it be done according to your faith and in the mighty name of Jesus!

Visit lauraharrissmith.com/blessings for the video blessing.

Your Endocrine System's A-list

Avoid bakery items, sugar, alcohol, refined carbs, wheat, trans fat; *stress*

Add almond flour, quinoa, avocado, walnuts, coconut oil, leafy greens

Allow flax and chia seeds, fish oil, iodine; vitamins A, B5, B6, D3; gingko, magnesium

Apply lavender, basil, lemon, geranium, clary sage, lemongrass oils

Anoint with oil daily and pray needed healing prayers and body system blessings

Ask your doctor or health care provider before making regimen changes

Your Endocrine System's Favorite . . .

Breakfast: salsa eggs (scrambled eggs with tomato, onion, cilantro, cayenne powder)

Lunch: yam fries with guacamole and cilantro; green salad with tomato, spinach, cucumbers, walnuts

Dinner: lentil soup with red onion, tomato, cayenne, cumin, turmeric; salad with olive oil and lemon

Snack: raspberries, blueberries, Brazil nuts, pistachios, cashews, almonds, pumpkin seeds, sunflower seeds

Testimony

"I could write you a book of all the many things God has done in just a few short days! The first night that I had these body system blessings, I began reading and fell asleep, and I woke up hours later in the recliner. Now, I know that sounds terrible, but for someone who has had insomnia for so long I can't remember, it was a gift! The next day, I picked up where I'd left off on the body system blessings and noticed that I had been reading the endocrine system blessing. I looked down and there were the last words I'd read before drifting off: "Your pineal gland makes the necessary melatonin for you to sleep well." I ran to my husband and we laughed. Surely it couldn't have worked so swiftly! Why do I still limit God's hands? I will continue to speak them out loud!" ~Saraha

After reading the blessings and prayers, send all testimonies large and small to healing@lauraharrissmith.com.

Endocrine System Healing Prayers

Adrenal Insufficiency (Adrenal Fatigue; Addison's Disease) Healing Prayer

Lord, I need Your energy. You created my body to be energized in numerous ways, an important one being through the hormones of adrenaline and cortisol. I have, through stress and a lack of proper rest, depleted almost my entire supply of both, and my body doesn't seem to want to create more. I need You to touch my adrenal glands and cause them to experience revival. I declare that my cortisol will rise sufficiently to help do its hundreds of jobs in my body, including maintaining my blood pressure and cardiovascular functions, balancing my insulin while breaking down sugars for energy, regulating my metabolism of carbohydrates, proteins and fats, and even assisting the pace at which my immune system's inflammatory response works. I declare that my hypothalamus will send the "releasing hormones" to my pituitary gland and that the response will be the release of just enough—but not too much—of my thyroid, adrenal, growth and reproductive hormones. Holy Spirit, come. Invigorate my body to thrive again and to be free from fatigue, unproductivity, secondary illnesses, depression, irritability and even the telltale salt cravings. Guide me to those who can help me make the life changes necessary so that I will not get myself in the same situation once You heal me. I am excited to abide by this chapter's A-list and aim for eight hours of sleep every night. "I can do all things through him who strengthens me" (Philippians 4:13). In Your name, Amen.

Cushing's Disease (Hypercortisolism) Healing Prayer

Lord, it seems my body wants to make too much cortisol, the result of which is all this fatigue, weight gain, excess sweating, excessive hair, high blood pressure, excessive hunger, muscle weakness, swelling and even potential osteoporosis. My midsection has become disproportionate, the fatty deposits between my shoulders have become pronounced, and I am ready to be done with the darkening skin and stretch marks, not to mention the mood swings. Holy Spirit, come. I refuse to be depressed, anxious or irritable. I will choose joy and health and youthfulness. I command my pituitary gland—in the name of Jesus—to stop releasing excess amounts of ACTH, and if the cause is a tumor growth (hyperplasia), then I ask You to heal and shrink it right now in Jesus' name. I know that cortisol is also released during stressful situations, so Father, please guide me in making the life changes necessary to walk in the divine health You intend for me. In Jesus' name, Amen.

Diabetes (Type 1 and Type 2) Healing Prayer

Blood sugar. Lord, these two words are not going to define and control my whole life! Right now I proclaim, first of all, that diabetes is just a name and that You, Jesus, have the name that is above all names. Whether it is type 1, where my pancreas needs a supernatural touch from You to function and create insulin again, or type 2, where my body needs my dietary help regulating the insulin that is being over- or underproduced, I assert my rights as a child of God to come to You for healing. In Your name I declare that my pancreas will do its job with perfection and that my insulin levels will be perfectly normal at all times. Holy Spirit, come. Diabetes, go, in Jesus' name! And any and all symptoms—body temperature changes, blurred vision, extreme hunger, darkening skin, fatigue, etc.—must go with it. My life will not be defined by shots and finger pricks and numbers. My life will, however, be defined by good choices and self-control and longevity. Father, help me abide by this chapter's A-list that will stabilize my body, meal by meal. "How sweet are Your words to my taste! Yes, sweeter than honey to my mouth!" (Psalm 119:103 NASB). Finally, Lord, I speak a blessing over any caretakers who have tended to my needs so diligently, including family, health professionals and even service animals. Through all these caretakers, You are with me in the waiting. In the name of Jesus I pray all of this by faith, Amen.

Growth Hormone Deficiency Healing Prayer

God, You created my body with the necessity to grow and heal, both of which are accomplished through the growth hormone somatotropin. My body has been deficient in that hormone, and as a result, my body is showing signs of the depletion. Holy Spirit, come. I ask You to touch my pituitary gland right now and cause it to release this growth hormone into my system, so that I can grow [for children], but most important, so that I can heal [for adults]. This hormone is vital for cell reproduction, without which it is next to impossible to recover from anything. I also need it in order to maintain the proper amounts of fat, muscle, tissue and bone in my body. Finally, with the presence of this hormone also comes a renewed sense of youthfulness, which I welcome wholeheartedly! Thank You in advance for this healing, Lord. "May you be strengthened with all power, according to His glorious might, for all endurance and patience with joy"(Colossians 1:11 HCSB). In Jesus' name, Amen.

Hyperthyroidism (Graves' Disease) Healing Prayer

Lord, surely You want my metabolism to move at a healthy pace so that my heart doesn't race, my muscles aren't weak, and my moods aren't so unpredictable. In Jesus' name I say goodbye to the fatigue, goiters, excess sweating, high blood pressure, heat intolerance, nervousness and anxiety! I ask You to touch my thyroid right now and stabilize the hormone it produces, so that my heart beats regularly without palpitations, my weight stabilizes, my eyes stop bulging, my bowel movements and menses [for women] return to normal, my hair grows back thick and lush, and my hands stop shaking. Let it be said of me, "So his hands were steady until the going down of the sun" (Exodus 17:12). Holy

Spirit, come. Guide me nutritionally through this chapter's A-list so that I can nourish my thyroid and maintain the miracle You are doing in it. In Jesus' name, Amen.

Hypoglycemia Healing Prayer

Jesus, I turn to You for healing from all blood sugar fluctuations that cause me to feel so weak and lifeless at times. I ask You to heal the hypoglycemia and all the symptoms that come with it, including the fainting, nausea, blurred vision, heart palpitations, clumsiness, tremors, slurred speech, headaches, excess sweating, light-headedness and shaking. I declare in Jesus' name that Psalm 62:2 is for me: "He only is my rock and my salvation, my stronghold; I shall not be greatly shaken" (NASB). God, stabilize my blood sugar, whether these crashes are reactions to diabetes treatments or just a lack of proper insulin regulation in my body. Holy Spirit, come. I surrender to you all fear, confusion, anxiety and irritability, and I ask for You to steady me—body, mind and spirit. You are my Healer, and it is in Your name I pray. Amen.

Hypopituitarism Healing Prayer

Lord, this tiny organ—my pituitary—is trying to cause big problems in my entire body, and I am asking You now for a healing touch. It is the master gland of my body, and I pray that You cause it to begin producing the hormones it was designed to produce, in the quantities in which You intended it to produce them. I trust You that I will not always have to deal with the anemia, hot flashes, weight loss, fatigue, difficult body temperature fluctuations, headaches, visual disturbances, hair loss, or even [if applicable] the infertility and decreased sex drive. I pray, Father, that should the cause be a tumor, You will dissolve it so that the hormones are no longer kept from their destinations. I do not want to be on medication for the rest of my life, and I ask You, O God, for a miracle. Holy Spirit, come. By healing this pea-sized organ in my body, You heal multiple other things, including my thyroid, adrenals, reproductive organs and the levels of the nine hormones my pituitary secretes. "Heal me, O LORD, and I shall be healed" (Jeremiah 17:14). In the name of Jesus I pray, Amen.

Hypothyroidism (Hashimoto's Disease) Healing Prayer

O Great Physician, only You can unravel what is going on in my body, and surely You stand ready to do just that. As my thyroid grows more and more sluggish, the rest of my body and metabolism seem to be coming to a screeching halt, but I am determined that You have an answer for me! I speak to my thyroid and tell it, "Wake up!" I command it, by the authority vested in me by You and Your healing Word, to produce sufficient thyroid hormone and to jump-start my metabolism. It will produce sufficient T3 (triiodothyronine) and T4 (thyroxine), which together will bring balance to my body temperature, metabolism and heart rate. The amounts secreted will be perfectly controlled by my TSH (thyroid stimulating hormone), which my pituitary gland will release with precision. With all this will come relief from all fatigue, lethargy, cold extremities, constipation, high cholesterol, low heart rate, sexual dysfunction, irregular uterine bleeding and more. And I even declare that I am about to get back my full head of hair, healthy nails and soft skin! Holy Spirit, come. Psalm 139:14 tells me that I am "fearfully and wonderfully made," so I am ready to feel wonderful again, God! Heal me and show me nutritionally how to maintain the miracle You are working in my body. In Jesus' name, Amen.

Metabolic Disorder (Insulin Resistance) Healing Prayer

Lord, help! There are so many things in my body that need fixing, that only You can name and heal them all. Yet I am confident that You will do just that. It seems that my blood sugar, weight and cholesterol all want to rise and create a cluster of conditions that have one name in common: metabolic disorder. Together they seek to cut my life short, but I proclaim long life over myself and say that I will not have a stroke, develop heart disease or have to live with diabetes. I am asking You, God, to heal me of all insulin resistance, unstable blood sugar levels, high triglycerides and all their symptoms, such as blurred vision, extreme thirst, weight gain (especially around the midsection), sluggish metabolism and more. Holy Spirit, come. I thank You for Your healing power and for the wisdom You are giving me through this chapter's A-list for using food as medicine and living long. Help me to get an exercise plan and to stay far ahead of the enemy, who seeks to cut my days short. I declare today that "I shall not die, but I shall live, and recount the deeds of the LORD" (Psalm 118:17). In Jesus' name I pray this, Amen.

Pancreatitis Healing Prayer

Jesus, I have been in pain and need You to touch my body and remove the inflammation in my pancreas. I declare that I will suffer with pancreatitis no more, nor will I suffer any of the fever, nausea, rapid pulse, abdominal pain or tenderness that accompanies it. I also reject any complications that would try to come from it, such as infections, kidney failure, diabetes, pseudocysts or even pancreatic cancer. Holy Spirit, come. As You touch my body, You are also gracing my mind with strategies for how to omit the foods that are inflaming my body, and how to incorporate the healing foods from this chapter's A-list that You have created for me so I can walk in divine health. I know that You do not want me suffering with this anymore, Lord. Revelation 21:4 says, "Neither shall there be any more pain: for the former things are passed away" (KJV), to which I say yes and amen! It is in Jesus' name I pray, Amen.

14

Circulatory System

Blood, All Vessels

Declaration

I am ready to receive any needed healing for my circulatory system and then do whatever it takes to walk in divine health. I know that God does not make me sick, and I ask Him right now to show me the root of my condition, whether it be physical, emotional or spiritual. I am ready to pray the prayer of faith, reverse the curse and unleash the blessing. By God's grace, I will watch my words and maintain my miracle or wait on God's perfect timing for healing. Amen!

Circulatory System Blessing

Right now, the blessing of the Lord is released upon your circulatory system to carry energized blood to every part of your body, bringing healing and better health where necessary. Your blood will carry fresh oxygen to body

Circulatory System

tissues and carry away waste products such as carbon dioxide. Your aorta, arteries, capillaries and veins are all connected properly, expand and retract where necessary and have no blockages. Your cholesterol is at a perfect level for your body's needs. Your superior vena cava and inferior vena cava bring blood from their delegated body sectors back to the chest and heart in perfect rhythm. I speak the Creator's wealth of wellness over all 60,000 miles of your circulatory system, which is enough to wrap around the world more than twice! And I declare that your blood itself—containing the plasma, white blood cells and platelets—is healthy, including the 5 million red blood cells in each drop. Let it be done according to your faith and in the mighty name of Jesus!

Visit lauraharrissmith.com/blessings for the video blessing.

Your Circulatory System's A-list

Avoid sugar, trans fats, excess salt (unless low blood pressure), canned meats, soda

Add garlic, oranges, lemons, nuts, salmon and cod, bell peppers; *exercise*

Allow ginkgo, fish oil, vitamin B3 (niacin), lycopene, resveratrol

Apply cyprus, ginger, black pepper, wintergreen, rosemary, lavender oils

Anoint with oil daily and pray needed healing prayers and body system blessings

Ask your doctor or health care provider before making regimen changes

Your Circulatory System's Favorite . . .

Breakfast: almonds; juice together citrus fruits and ginger root with a dash of cayenne powder

Lunch: roasted broccoli with olive oil, slivered almonds, pink salt; salad with veggies, olive oil, ACV

Dinner: roasted Brussels sprouts with olive oil; salad with walnuts; cauliflower rice; salmon or chicken

Snack: citrus fruits, nuts, strawberries, blueberries, 70–80 percent cocoa organic dark chocolate, green tea

Testimony

"I have been praying the circulatory blessing over myself, particularly for my blood cholesterol levels. My levels had been stuck in the mid-200s for several years. I began eating the healthy foods on Laura's A-list, but what happened transpired so fast that it had to be the supernatural work of the body system blessings, because after only weeks I got new labs back and my cholesterol is down to 185!" ~Larry

After reading the blessings and prayers, send all testimonies large and small to healing@lauraharrissmith.com.

Circulatory System Healing Prayers

Anemia Healing Prayer

Lord, I am tired of feeling tired. In Your name I turn to You and ask for healing. Please reproduce my red blood cells at a supernatural rate, Lord, because at present there are not enough of them to carry proper oxygen to my body's tissues. Jesus, You do not want me weak, so I resist the weakness. Joel 3:10 says, "Let the weak say, I am strong!" (KJV). That will be my anthem. I refuse all forms of anemia, including aplastic anemia, autoimmune hemolytic anemia, thalassemia and even sickle cell anemia. I trade in the fatigue for strength, the dizziness for steadiness, the shortness of breath for regular breaths and this fast heartbeat for a normal one. I also thank You that You are delivering me from the headaches, brittle nails, pale skin and overall malaise. "I am strong!" Holy Spirit, come. Give me an appetite for the iron-rich foods on this chapter's A-list so that I might stay strong at all times. I pray and declare this in Your name, Jesus. Amen.

Arteriosclerosis and Atherosclerosis Healing Prayer

Lord, it seems that my blood vessels are trying to stiffen and become thick, thereby restricting the flow of blood, nutrients and oxygen to the rest of my body. Reverse this hardening of my arteries, Lord, and along with healing the arteriosclerosis, please also heal and prevent any atherosclerosis, which is the buildup of plaque (fats and cholesterol) in my arteries. Help me abide by this chapter's A-list to avoid plaque buildup, so that I might not have dangerous blockage or, worse, have the plaque burst and cause a blood clot that triggers a heart attack or stroke. Holy Spirit, come. I give You any symptoms of leg pain when walking (claudication), chest pain or pressure (angina), and TIA symptoms and temporary loss of vision or slurred speech, which would mean that the arteries leading to my brain were blocked. I expect to feel better, eat better and get better, with Your help. May John 7:38 be said of me and of this healing You are doing in the blood flow of my body: "Out of his heart will flow rivers . . ." In Jesus' name, Amen.

Blood Clots (Thrombus) Healing Prayer

Father, somewhere in the hidden places of my veins, the flow of my blood has come into contact with substances in my skin or blood that have begun to clump together in a chain reaction and form clots. Only You know how many clots there are and what dangerous locations they are in. Lord, thank You for the way You created my blood to clot when needed (as in case of an injury or cut, where blood flow needs to stop). But in this case, I need You to stop the clotting. I speak to the waxy cholesterol plaques that seem to have formed in my arteries, and I declare that they will dissolve, but not burst and lead to a stroke. I commit to eating the right foods on this chapter's A-list so I can cooperate with what You are doing in my body, maintain my miracle and not lose ground. I proclaim that my blood will flow freely and not pool in my vessels or allow the platelets to stick together. I will not have proteins that clot together or long strands of fibrin that get tangled up with my platelets and form serious clotting. Holy Spirit, come. My blood will flow unobstructed, as God created it to do. Thank You, Lord, that Isaiah 57:14 says, "Remove every obstruction from my people's way." I claim that for my circulatory system in Jesus' name, Amen.

Blood Disorders Healing Prayer

Lord, Leviticus 17:11 says, "Life is in the blood" (CEV), so the importance of my circulatory system's health is vital in order for me to stay alive. Almighty God, whether this blood disease is attacking my red blood cells, white blood cells, platelets or plasma, I trust You to heal it right now in the name of Your Son. Holy Spirit, come. I resist every blood disease, including the ones that come against red blood cell health [see the anemia healing prayer in this chapter and the malaria prayer in chapter 24], and those diseases that come against white blood cells [see the lymphoma and leukemia prayers in chapter 24], or disorders that affect my platelets, such as essential thrombocytosis, thrombocytopenia, idiopathic thrombocytopenic purpura, and heparin-induced thrombocytopenia. I also ask for protection from anything that would seek to harm my blood plasma [see the hemophilia and deep vein thrombosis prayers that follow]. Thank You, Father, for healing me and keeping my blood flowing freely for perfect health. In Jesus' name I pray, Amen.

Deep Vein Thrombosis (DVT or VTE) Healing Prayer

In the name of Jesus I declare that I will not develop blood clots at all [see the blood clots healing prayer in this chapter], but that I especially will not have blood clots form in the deep veins of my body, particularly my legs. Heal me, O God, and safely dissolve any clots that have tried to form in my deepest veins, keeping me safe from them traveling throughout my body and causing pulmonary embolisms. I thank You that there will be no more swelling in my extremities, or cramping, soreness, tenderness or discoloration, or warm sensations over my veins. Holy Spirit, come. I will get moving and find exercise that I enjoy so that my circulatory system can constantly be flowing and cleansed. Invigorate my blood, God. I receive Your healing right now. "Let thy vein be blessed" (Proverbs 5:18 DRA). In Jesus' name, Amen.

Edema Healing Prayer

God, I am told that the tiniest capillaries in my body are leaking fluid and causing all this swelling. Would You touch me now and heal this seepage and strengthen my veins? I praise You in advance, knowing that whether this was caused by too much salt, pregnancy, sitting too long or even PMS, You can bring me relief. And Lord, if it should be telling me that there is a more serious issue such as congestive heart failure, cirrhosis, kidney damage, severe protein deficiency or lymphatic system issues, I receive Your healing right now for them all. Holy Spirit, come. I declare my deliverance from stiffness, difficulty walking, any blisters due to swelling, chest pain, shortness of breath, decreased blood circulation and stretched or itchy skin. I ask You to replace it all with relief and healing. "You give them relief" (Psalm 94:13 NLT). In Jesus' name I pray and receive, Amen.

Hematoma Healing Prayer

Lord, this collection of blood outside my blood vessel(s) is painful and dangerous. Heal this hematoma, Jesus, regardless of its location. Touch the hidden areas inside the walls of my veins, blood vessels, arteries and capillaries, and dry up any leakage where my blood has traveled to areas where it does not belong. Places that have caused large areas of bruising and swelling, or even tiny dot hematomas—heal them all, Jesus. And I declare that I will not suffer any headaches or confusion, back pain or abdominal pain, nail loss or nail pain, bladder or bowel incontinence, or bruises and seizures. I declare that my blood will flow without clotting and stay where it is supposed to, and that the walls of my veins and tiny passageways in my circulatory system will be strong and secure, according to the healing promised to me in Your Word. Holy Spirit, come. It will be said of me, "His [or her] heart pumps God's Word like blood through his [or her] veins" (Psalm 37:30–31 MESSAGE). It is in the name of Jesus I pray, Amen.

Hemophilia Healing Prayer

Lord, You created the body's blood to be able to clot when necessary so that we do not bleed excessively, but my body has not been cooperating. Jesus, I ask You to touch my circulatory system and cause its blood to be perfect in all ways, including in its ability to clot when I am injured or cut. I call for relief from the bruises, endless bleeding, blood in the urine, nosebleeds, rectal bleeding, joint pain, severe blood loss, weakness and prolonged periods. "Then this one with human appearance touched me again and strengthened me" (Daniel 10:18 NASB). Holy Spirit, come. I receive Your strengthening touch right now in the name of the Son, Jesus. Amen.

Hemorrhage Healing Prayer

Lord, there are so many things that could be causing this hemorrhaging, but I tell the blood to dry up right now in the name of Jesus. Whatever the cause—a burst vessel, a vitamin K deficiency, a bowel obstruction or acute bronchitis—I command it to stop in Your healing name. If it is something more serious—brain trauma, leukemia, lung cancer, prolonged menstrual bleeding or liver disease—I declare that You are still able to heal the underlying condition and cause me to be strengthened right now. If the blood loss is substantial or if there is an injury, then show me whom to reach out to right now, Father, to assist me. Holy Spirit, come. I know that You are with me as I recover, and like the woman who touched You in Luke 8:43–44, I am ready for Your touch: "In the crowd that day there was a woman who for twelve years had been afflicted with hemorrhages. She had spent every penny she had on doctors but not one had been able to help her. She slipped in from behind and touched the edge of Jesus' robe. At that very moment her hemorrhaging stopped" (MESSAGE). In Jesus' name I pray and receive, Amen.

High Cholesterol (Hypercholesterolemia) Healing Prayer

Lord, high cholesterol has no symptoms, so I was surprised by this blood test result from my doctor. I now ask You to show me what I am doing that elevated my cholesterol, such as a poor diet, lack of exercise, smoking, being overweight or not managing my blood sugar. And then give me a strategy to lower it. I know I need cholesterol to make my hormones and cell membranes, but, Lord, get it to the level that is safest for me and for my body's needs. In the name of Jesus I say that as I cooperate with God in my healing, the flow of blood in my arteries will not be restricted and will not lead to chest pain, heart attacks or strokes. And, Lord, while I am lowering my bad cholesterol (low-density lipoprotein, or LDL), help me eat from the foods on this chapter's A-list and raise my good cholesterol (high-density lipoprotein, or HDL). Holy Spirit, come. I am committed to good health and won't ask You to help me if I am not willing to help myself. Grant me the self-discipline to make these changes. "But the fruit of the Spirit is . . . self-control" (Galatians 5:22–23). In Jesus' name I pray, Amen.

Mitral Valve Prolapse Healing Prayer

In the name of Jesus I command my heartbeat to stabilize. I declare that the leaflets of my heart's mitral valve will stop bulging into my heart's upper left chamber during its contraction. I speak health over the valve, and in Your name, Father, I receive Your healing and declare that the blood will not run backward into my left atrium and result in mitral valve regurgitation. Holy Spirit, come. I thank You that You are healing me from the shortness of breath, dizziness, irregular heartbeat and blood pressure, palpitations, fatigue, murmur and chest pressure. I thank You that my circulatory system and cardiovascular system are working in perfect symmetry to provide the energy and health that my body needs to thrive, one perfect heartbeat at a time. I receive Psalm 57:7 for myself: "My heart is steadfast, O God, my heart is steadfast! I will sing and make melody!" In the name of Jesus I pray, Amen.

Peripheral Artery Disease Healing Prayer

Jesus, only You can see into each blood vessel of my body and clear the narrowing in each one. I ask You now especially to clear those going to my extremities—my legs—so that I might be out of this leg pain and total body danger. Remove from me the claudication (leg pain), leg numbness, cold feet and legs, weak pulse in legs, hair loss or slow hair growth on the legs, slower growing toenails, slow-healing foot sores, discoloration, and erectile dysfunction [in males]. Holy Spirit, come. Help my rest at night to be peaceful, and please ease the ischemic pain that disrupts my sleep. Remove the fatty deposits entirely from my circulatory system, God, and give me the desire for better foods and more exercise. "Therefore my heart is glad, and my whole being rejoices; my flesh also dwells secure" (Psalm 16:9). Let it be so. In Jesus' name I pray, Amen.

Sickle Cell Disease Healing Prayer

Father, I need You to touch my red blood cells. They have become misshapen and have begun to die early. This shortage of red blood cells has resulted in an anemia that has left me weak, but I know that You intend healing for me. Break this inherited physical curse, Lord, and keep it from the legacy I leave, too. I ask You to heal me from the dizziness, paleness, jaundice, sudden chest pain, inflamed fingers and toes, joint pain, fatigue, low blood oxygen, blood in my urine and even delayed development. I also declare that my life expectancy is not shortened, but that I will fulfill every day God has ordained for me on this earth. Holy Spirit, come. I proclaim right now in the name of Jesus that my circulatory system and its blood cells are healthy and strong, just like my heart. "O LORD, you hear the desire of the afflicted; you will strengthen their heart" (Psalm 10:17).

Stroke Healing Prayer

Lord, I've been told that the blood supply to my brain was interrupted and that my brain tissue was deprived of oxygen and nutrients. A stroke. First, I surrender my fear to You and thank You for saving my life, for I know that I could be in a much worse situation than I am now. But I have been left with much to overcome, and right now I declare that You are my Healer and that I will fully recover. I pray for my muscular system, that You would heal it of any paralysis and help me with my balance, coordination, walking, swallowing, overactive reflexes, stiffness, and any numbness in my face, arms or legs. Holy Spirit, come. Touch my sensory system so that I might be able to see without blurred vision, double vision or sudden visual loss, and so that I might be able to speak clearly without slurred speech or loss of understanding. Heal the pins and needles and reduced sensation of touch, and rejuvenate me from the fatigue, vertigo, dizziness, headache and mental confusion. Touch my brain in the Broca's and Wernicke's areas that help me speak and comprehend, and I command all visual problems to cease. And finally, Lord, restore my circulatory system so that the blood supply to my brain is never reduced or compromised again, and bring health to my entire body. "O Lord my God, I cried to you for help, and you have healed me" (Psalm 30:2). I declare it to be so in the name of Jesus, Amen.

Varicose Veins Healing Prayer

Jesus, it is the desire of my heart for these ugly, painful varicose veins to be healed. I am asking as Your child that You would touch my circulatory system and reshape the veins that are so twisted and bulging in my legs (or face). Holy Spirit, come. Reduce the swelling, and remove the constant bruising, itching, heaviness, discoloration and discomfort. Shrink the spider veins, too, that are closer to the surface. And Lord, most importantly, cause the blood in my body to circulate better so that the blood in my legs can defy gravity and return blood to my heart. May it be said of me that my "veins are filled with nourishment" (Job 21:24 AMPC). In the name of Jesus I pray all of this, Amen.

15

Cardiovascular System

*Heart, Blood Vessels:
Arteries, Capillaries, Veins*

Declaration

I am ready to receive any needed healing for my cardio-vascular system and then do whatever it takes to walk in divine health. I know that God does not make me sick, and I ask Him right now to show me the root of my condition, whether it be physical, emotional or spiritual. I am ready to pray the prayer of faith, reverse the curse and unleash the blessing. By God's grace, I will watch my words, maintain my miracle or wait on God's perfect timing for healing. Amen!

Cardiovascular System Blessing

God's promise of health begins in your heart right now, and I release the blessing of divine Cardiovascular System health upon this life force in your chest that beats more than 100,000 times per day. An average heartbeat of 80 beats per minute for a lifetime of 80 years means that your heart will beat more than 3 billion times. Yours will not skip a beat! Using the circulatory system's 60,000-mile network of vessels, capillaries, arteries, etc., your heart is pumping the necessary oxygen and nutrient-rich, energized blood throughout your entire body to sustain perfect health for you. Your blood pressure is stable, and in your heart there is no fluttering, racing, discomfort, shortness of breath, light-headedness, fainting or attacks. Let it be done according to your faith and in the mighty name of Jesus!

Visit lauraharrissmith.com/blessings for the video blessing.

Your Cardiovascular System's A-list

Avoid sugar, refined carbs, margarine, processed meats, bacon, trans fats

Add walnuts, almonds, green tea, citrus, legumes, tomato, flaxseed; *cardio*

Allow Niacin (B3), folate, calcium, magnesium taurate, lycopene, fish oil

Apply basil, ginger, cypress, helichrysum, cassia, clove, marjoram oils

Anoint with oil daily and pray needed healing prayers and body system blessings

Ask your doctor or health care provider before making regimen changes

Your Cardiovascular System's Favorite . . .

Breakfast: steel-cut oatmeal with stevia or Swerve, cinnamon, walnuts, blueberries

Lunch: oven-roasted beet chips with pink salt; asparagus; organic steroid-free chicken or salmon with garlic

Dinner: spaghetti squash with garlic and tomato sauce; broccoli; salad with nuts, olive oil, lemon

Snack: blueberries, red bell peppers, edamame, cucumbers, almonds, watermelon, pumpkin seeds, green tea, 70–80 percent cocoa organic dark chocolate

Testimony

"After reading Laura's book and putting her food suggestions into practice, within a month test results showed my cholesterol, triglycerides and LDL went down and my HDL improved. Also, the nodule on the right side of my thyroid decreased in size, which was noted on the medical report. My blood pressure medication was reduced in dosage, with the plan being no longer to need it. All of these are important factors for a healthy cardiovascular system. Although results were positive and I felt much better, I eventually slipped back into old habits. Because of my bad choices, I ended up in the ER with heart palpitations. My heart was beating up to 150 times per minute, putting me at serious risk of having a stroke. Surgery was required. It was an eye-opener. I am back to following Laura's food suggestions and eating heart-healthy foods. My most recent cardiologist follow-up indicated positive results. I was taken off three out of five medications, with the goal to be rid of all medications. Most of all, not only is my heart healing physically, but by praying and believing, I am healing emotionally and spiritually. All three are equally necessary for overall health. I truly believe that it is not just about living longer, but about living better. God bless Laura, her team and each of you!" ~Marianne

> After reading the blessings and prayers, send all testimonies large and small to healing@lauraharrissmith.com.

Cardiovascular System Healing Prayers

Aortic Aneurysm Healing Prayer

Jesus, please touch my heart right now and remove the dangerous bulge in the wall of my aorta. I need this major blood vessel that carries blood from my heart to the rest of my body to be healthy. Whether the bulge is fusiform (tube shaped) or saccular (round), I know that You can cause this bulge to be gone in an instant, without any danger to my heart itself. Lord, if this is an abdominal aortic aneurysm, then please mend this delicate highway passing through my abdomen. If it is a thoracic aortic aneurysm and passes through my chest cavity, please touch that part near my heart and forever protect me from having aortic disease. Holy Spirit, come. I declare that there will be no aortic dissections, ruptures or tears and that the walls of my aorta will be strong all the days of my life. This is a delicate area to repair and human hands could falter, but You are the Great Physician and know exactly what's wrong and how to fix it. Lord, "examine my heart" (Psalm 26:2 NIV). In Jesus' name, Amen.

Angina Healing Prayer

Jesus, I am asking You to heal this pain in my chest, which has been diagnosed as angina. I say "enough" of the squeezing, pressure, nausea, fatigue, shortness of breath, sweating and dizziness. I also know that this is just a symptom of a larger issue, which is coronary artery disease (arteriosclerosis), so heal me of that, too, Father, helping me abide by this chapter's A-list for clearer arteries. Whether this is stable angina (occurring only when I exert myself, walk up stairs or exercise), or unstable angina (occurring unexpectedly and even when at rest), I command it to go right now, and I receive Your healing, Jesus. And Lord, protect and heal me from the worst, variant angina, and of course from a heart attack itself. Holy Spirit, come. I know that You are watching over me and I can be at peace, as can my entire cardiovascular system. Let it not be with me as Psalm 38, verse 10 says: "My heart throbs; my strength fails me, and the light of my eyes—it also has gone from me." Instead, I make verse 22 my cry: "Make haste to help me, O Lord, my salvation!" I agree and pray this in Jesus' name, Amen.

Arrhythmia (Tachycardia or Bradycardia) Healing Prayer

Lord, I need You to synchronize my cardiovascular system with my nervous system and cause the electrical impulses that coordinate my heartbeats to keep better time. Whether my heart is beating too fast (tachycardia) or too slow (bradycardia), please heal it now and stabilize its rhythm. And while I know that not all irregular heartbeats mean that I have heart disease, if You do see anything wrong within my cardiovascular or circulatory systems, I ask You to repair it, and I receive Your healing right now. Lord, thank You for putting an end to the chest pain, irregular heartbeat, shortness of breath, fainting, sweating, dizziness, chest flutters and, most of all, the fear and dread that I am going to die of a heart attack. Holy Spirit, come. I will listen to Your wisdom. If you choose for me a progressive healing that involves medical assistance, then grace me to follow my doctor's orders and to make wise nutritional decisions that will help You answer My prayers. "Wait for the Lord; be strong, and let your heart take courage; wait for the Lord!" (Psalm 27:14.) It is in Jesus' name I pray, Amen.

Atrial Fibrillation (AFib/AF) Healing Prayer

God, in addition to the arrhythmia prayer I also prayed, I ask You please to heal me of the most dangerous version of tachycardia, which is where the top two chambers of my heart (the atria) beat out of rhythm with the bottom two chambers (the ventricles) and cause my heart to receive blood back from the rest of my body too quickly. I receive Your healing touch right now, by faith, to synchronize all four chambers and the electrical impulses of my heartbeat so that I might never again experience the dizziness, palpitations, shortness of breath, fatigue, weakness and inability to exercise. And if the arrhythmia is the result of thyroid or blood sugar issues or any other primary cause, please heal me of that, too. Should it be a reaction to medicine or food, please show me what it is, so that I might abstain. Holy Spirit, come. Protect me from any future dangers AFib could lead to, such as blood clots, heart failure, stroke or other complications. "His heart is steady; he will not be afraid" (Psalm 112:8). I receive Your healing right now in the name of Jesus, Amen.

Cardiomyopathy (Myocardial Disease) Healing Prayer

Jesus, just as You have touched my spiritual heart and made it new, I know You can also touch my physical heart and do the same. My heart muscle needs healing from its inability to pump blood to the rest of my body, and I know that this is a small thing for You to accomplish for me. Whether the issue is that my heart's main pumping chamber—the left ventricle—has become enlarged and cannot effectively pump blood (dilated cardiomyopathy), or that my left ventricle heart muscle has become abnormally thick (hypertrophic cardiomyopathy), please heal me now, Lord. And if it is just that my heart muscle has become less elastic and more rigid overall (restrictive cardiomyopathy), or that my lower right heart chamber—the right ventricle—has developed scar tissue and become irregular (arrhythmogenic right ventricular dysplasia), then I ask You to touch that and my entire cardiovascular system right now and make it whole. Holy Spirit, come. Show me where I am at risk, whether it be from genetics, obesity, long-term high blood pressure, diabetes, drug or alcohol use or anything else, and help me stick to the advice on this chapter's A-list. "The LORD is my strength and my shield; in him my heart trusts, and I am helped; my heart exults, and with my song I give thanks to him" (Psalm 28:7). In the name of Jesus, Amen.

Congestive Heart Failure Healing Prayer

Lord, a diagnosis of congestive heart failure is scary, but I know that You are with me and that You have sustained my life thus far. I declare, in the name of Jesus, that my heart will not fail to pump blood through my body into each place the blood is supposed to go and back. My heart will be strong, and I will work daily to make it stronger through diet and exercise. Lord, I give You all the chest pain, dizziness, loss of appetite, fatigue, cough and phlegm, and weight gain. I also declare that I am free from the palpitations, difficulty breathing when lying down, water retention, swollen feet, bloating and excess urination at night. Take them all away and make me whole. Lord, I don't want to have a heart transplant because I know that means that someone else must die for me to live, and Your Son has already paid that price for me. But my treatment is in Your hands, and if You should choose a healing remedy over a miracle, then I will submit to Your plan. Holy Spirit, come. I receive Psalm 69:32 for myself: "You who seek God, let your heart revive" (NASB). Amen! In Your name, Jesus!

Endocarditis Healing Prayer

Father, I come to You with this diagnosis of endocarditis and ask You to touch the three layers of my heart: the outer epicardium layer, the middle myocardium layer, and the innermost endocardium layer. Evidently, this endocardium layer is inflamed, along with my heart valves. I am not sure which came first—a damaged nerve or bacteria in my bloodstream that attached to it— but I need You to heal both right now. I know You are my Healer and can do more than the antibiotics can do, and with much less damage to my digestive and immune systems, so please touch me now. Holy Spirit, come. Take away all the symptoms of fatigue, chills, shortness of breath, joint pain, red spots under the skin, and sweating. Let me feel Your strength and peace, day and night.

"And let the peace of Christ rule in your hearts" (Colossians 3:15). In the name of Jesus I pray, Amen.

Heart Attack Intervention Prayer and Recovery Healing Prayers

Note: This prayer is to be prayed over someone only after first calling 911.

"My anguish, my anguish! I writhe in pain! Oh the walls of my heart! My heart is beating wildly; I cannot keep silent, for I hear the sound of the trumpet, the alarm of war" (Jeremiah 4:19). Father, in the name of Jesus, I command the spirit of death to go. I declare _____ will live and not die, and I command the cardiovascular system and circulatory system to be at peace and to begin functioning with complete accuracy and perfect rhythm. Spirit of life, come! Spirit of death, you are defeated, and now new life and healing will take your place. In Jesus' name, Amen.

Note: This prayer is for recovery after a heart attack.

God, thank You for saving my life! Now more than ever, I know that You left me here on earth for a purpose, and I praise You. Jesus, continue to heal my heart, valves and every other part of my cardiovascular and circulatory systems. Holy Spirit, come. Help me stick to the advice on this chapter's A-list. I do not want to beg You for healing in my heart and then undermine Your miracles by undoing them with my food choices. Thank You for my life and for new grace to live it. In Your name I pray and thank You, Amen!

Hypertension (High Blood Pressure) Healing Prayer

Jesus, I know there are no real symptoms of high blood pressure, but I also know that when checking mine, it has had a tendency to be high lately. I need my systolic (the number on top) to be between 90 and 120, and I need my diastolic (the bottom number) to be between 60 and 80. God, I need a strategy from You for how to correct my current numbers. I can ask You to heal me, but if those healing prayers leave my mouth and then I stuff unhealthy foods in it and expect to be well, I am deceived. Holy Spirit, come. Convict me to abide by the advice in this chapter's A-list, to exercise regularly and to achieve my healthiest weight. Help me with the weight loss, Lord! And I also ask for Your revelation on how I can better manage the stress in my life, or remove it entirely. You are my Great Physician, Lord, and I am Your patient. I know that Psalm 22:26 is for me: "The afflicted shall eat and be satisfied; those who seek him shall praise the LORD! May your hearts live forever!" I pray it in Jesus' name, Amen.

Pericarditis Healing Prayer

In the name of Jesus I proclaim that the saclike membrane surrounding my heart—my pericardium—is perfect and healed. It will no longer be swollen or irritated, and any infection present is leaving right now, as I pray. Take with it, Father, the stabbing chest pain, left shoulder or neck pain, fatigue, fever, pressure and shortness of breath. I know this is not a serious condition, but if it becomes chronic, then it could take weeks or months to heal. With Your Help, O Great God, I will beat those odds, and do so without surgery. Holy Spirit, come. You are my Healer! "I have trusted in your steadfast love; my heart shall rejoice in your salvation" (Psalm 13:5). In the name of Jesus I ask it all, Amen.

16

Respiratory System

*Lungs, Nose, Pharynx, Larynx,
Trachea, Bronchi, Alveoli*

Declaration

I am ready to receive any needed healing for my respiratory system and then do whatever it takes to walk in divine health. I know that God does not make me sick, and I ask Him right now to show me the root of my condition, whether it be physical, emotional or spiritual. I am ready to pray the prayer of faith, reverse the curse and unleash the blessing. By God's grace, I will watch my words, maintain my miracle or wait on God's perfect timing for healing. Amen!

Respiratory System Blessing

Take the deepest breath you can and get ready for rejuvenation to your entire respiratory system. I speak **Respiratory System** healing and wholeness over the entire system, from your nose to your lungs, in the mighty name of Jesus. I release the blessing of clear nasal passages and a healthy mouth with which to take in adequate oxygen. Your throat is free from infection because your tonsils have done their job; your larynx is free of any blockages, and the pathways are perfectly clear to your windpipe (trachea). There is no inflammation in your bronchial tubes, bronchioles or alveoli, and your lungs will expand and compress without restriction, pain or collapsing. There will be just enough mucus present to keep your lungs moist and to stop viruses, dust and bacteria, but not enough to cause irritation and constant coughing. Whether inhaling or exhaling, your lungs are being restored to perfect condition right now, and you can expect to have increased energy, heartier laughter and better rest. Let it be done according to your faith, and in the mighty name of Jesus!

Visit lauraharrissmith.com/blessings for the video blessing.

Your Respiratory System's A-list

Avoid dairy, excess salt, sodas, sugar, fruit juice, wine, eggs, cold cuts

Add warm foods like bone broth, soups, teas; citrus, pomegranate; *laughter*

Allow fish oil, zinc; vitamins B6, B12, C, E; folate, quercetin, bromelain

Apply eucalyptus, lemon, peppermint, tea tree, lavender, rosemary oils

Anoint with oil daily and pray needed healing prayers and body system blessings

Ask your doctor or health care provider before making regimen changes

Your Respiratory System's Favorite . . .

Breakfast: smoothie—1 kiwi, 1 orange, ½ cup papaya, 1 inch ginger root, ½ teaspoon cayenne, 1 to 2 cups water

Lunch: leafy green salad and lentil stew with kale, onion, tomatoes, turmeric, cayenne, garlic

Dinner: broccoli, Laura's curry chicken or tofu (at lauraharrissmith.com/recipes), cauliflower rice

Snack: dark berries, apples, citrus fruits, apricots, pumpkin seeds, sunflower seeds, nut butters, nuts, hummus with cayenne, cucumbers

Testimony

"I have suffered from asthma since I was a small child. When I would take deep breaths or help take groceries out of the car, I would have a hard time breathing, and it would keep me from working out! I read the respiratory body blessing over myself on Saturday night, and Sunday I helped get the groceries out of the car and was not out of breath! Also, I have suffered from migraines and neck pain for several years, but when I read the nervous system body blessing, I felt heat and a hand on the back of my neck! It felt as if someone were taking a heating pad to my neck to help with my migraine and neck pain. I haven't had a headache since!" ~Clark

> After reading the blessings and prayers, send all testimonies large and small to healing@lauraharrissmith.com.

Respiratory System Healing Prayers

Asthma Healing Prayer

Jesus, You put the breath in my lungs on the day I was born, and I know that You do not want that breath stolen. I ask You to clear my passageways and heal this asthma, Lord. I give You the breathing difficulties, chest pain and wheezing, and along with those, I ask You to take away the anxiety, fear, heart palpitations and sleep interferences. God, I want to be able to exercise, walk, run and live an active life without fear of suffocation or constantly being short of breath. In return, I receive the ability to breathe deeply at a normal rate and, more importantly, never to have to think about breath again! Holy Spirit, come. I give You praise for this miracle You are going to do in my body. "I bless GOD every chance I get; my lungs expand with his praise. I live and breathe GOD" (Psalm 34:1–2 MESSAGE). In the name of Jesus I pray, Amen.

Bronchitis Healing Prayer

God, I need a respiratory miracle today. Please heal me of this chronic coughing, or at the very least, make it productive so that it rids my lungs of the congestion inside. Decrease the inflammation that lines the bronchiole tubes, and please heal me of the cold symptoms as well—the runny nose, postnasal drip, headache, sore throat and shortness of breath. I ask for relief from the chest pressure, fatigue, sleeping difficulties and all this phlegm! Holy Spirit, come. Thank You for making healing foods for my respiratory system that expedite my healing. I receive Your invitation to make the changes necessary for better health, adhering to this chapter's A-list nutritional advice. "Thus says God, the LORD, who created the heavens and stretched them out, who spread out the earth and what comes from it, who gives breath to the people on it and spirit to those who walk in it" (Isaiah 42:5). I ask it all in Your name, Jesus. Amen.

COPD (Chronic Obstructive Pulmonary Disease) Healing Prayer

Lord, I am turning to You for healing today in my lungs. I believe that right now You are taking this inflammation and calming it—even reversing it. Passageways are opening up and my breathing is becoming easier, in Jesus' name. I declare that I will not always struggle with wheezing, shortness of breath, chest pressure, constant respiratory infections and chronic cough. And I know doctors say that the damage caused to the lungs by COPD is irreversible, but You are the Great Physician and I know You can prove this untrue. So, Lord, I thank You for my healing, and I look forward to running, exercising, climbing stairs, playing with the young children in my life, and not having to live on steroids or in constant fear of getting too far away from my rescue inhalers. I look forward to not even being dependent on oxygen machine use. Holy Spirit, come. This is my year to thrive. Convict me to adhere to the advice on this chapter's A-list and to refrain from those things harming my lungs (such as smoking). "With your very own hands you formed me; now breathe your wisdom over me so I can understand you" (Psalm 119:73, MESSAGE). I ask it all in Your name, Jesus. Amen.

Cystic Fibrosis Healing Prayer

Lord, the diagnosis and lifestyle of living with cystic fibrosis have been difficult. I know You have been my Helper, and I thank You. But, God, I turn to You now for healing, knowing that only You can do this respiratory miracle in my body. Holy Spirit, come. Please heal the cells that are producing the mucus, sweat and digestive juices so that the fluids no longer become sticky and thick. Please clear all the passageways, tubes and ducts from the constant plugging, and bring protection from the common occurrences of pneumonia and acute bronchitis. I declare freedom from the diarrhea, fatty stools and constipation and ask for healing from the pulmonary hypertension, wheezing, infections and sinusitis. Lord, bring healing all over, including to any delayed development or slow growth. Bring energy instead of fatigue, weight gain instead of weight loss, activity instead of inability to exercise and most of all, no more blood loss when coughing. "You saw my pain, you disarmed my tormentors, you didn't leave me in their clutches but gave me room to breathe" (Psalm 31:6–7 MESSAGE). I ask it all in the name of Jesus. Amen.

Emphysema Healing Prayer

Father, I know You can do a miracle in my respiratory system. I am weary of being short of breath, and of the constant inflammation in my bronchial tubes. The inner walls of my air sacs have become weak and possibly ruptured, creating larger air spaces and reducing the surface area of my lungs. Thus, the amount of oxygen that can reach my bloodstream has been reduced. Holy Spirit, come. I seek You for healing of the resulting fatigue, shortness of breath and my inability to stay focused and be mentally alert. Lead me to work and home environments with clearer air and less indoor and outdoor pollution, and no secondhand smoke. And of course, there will be no firsthand smoking of any kind for me. Bless my lungs with new, vibrant health; I know my youth will be renewed like the eagle's. "Don't grieve God. Don't break his heart. His Holy Spirit, moving and breathing in you, is the most intimate part of your life, making you fit for himself. Don't take such a gift for granted" (Ephesians 4:30 MESSAGE). In Jesus' name, Amen.

Pneumonia (and Legionnaires' Disease) Healing Prayer

In the name of Jesus, I ask for healing from this pneumonia. Touch the air sacs in my lungs, empty them of the fluid or pus, Lord, and bring peace to the inflammation and an end to the infection. Holy Spirit, come. I thank You that as this infection leaves, the fever, chills, fatigue and loss of appetite will leave with it. Where I was short of breath, I will now be able to breathe deeply. Where I had no energy, I will now be active. Where I had no appetite, I will now be able to nourish myself with healing foods. Thank You for bringing an end to the sharp chest pains, chronic coughing and wheezing. You are my Great Physician and the only one who can heal. "Let everything that has breath praise the LORD! Praise the LORD!" (Psalm 150:6). I ask it in the name of Jesus. Amen.

Pneumothorax Healing Prayer

Note: In 2013, God miraculously healed me of a pneumothorax in minutes. I had taken a strange fall into a rod-and-glass iron table, broken a rib and punctured a lung, and it began collapsing. The pain was unlike anything I had ever experienced, even childbirth. After three days of immobility, I cried out to God in agony. Within minutes, the pain left and my mobility returned. The next day, an X-ray showed the rib was no longer broken and the collapsing lung had completely reinflated. Please let this build your faith about what our God is capable of! I will lead you in the exact prayer I prayed then:

Dear Lord, I am in great need of Your healing. Only You can touch my lung(s); seal and reinflate the collapsed lung. Lord, if You will do this for me, which I know You want to, I will shout it from the rooftops and give glory to Your name. Holy Spirit, come.

And then I wrote in lipstick on my bedroom mirror an excerpt from Ezekiel 37:9, which became part of my prayer:

"Prophesy to the breath; prophesy, son of man, and say to the breath, Thus says the Lord God: Come from the four winds, O breath, and breathe . . ." In Jesus' name I pray, Amen.

Pulmonary Embolism (PE) Healing Prayer

Lord, I realize the danger that these blood clots present to my lungs. I am asking You to dissolve them with no further danger to my body. Heal me of the chest pain, leg pain and swelling, especially in the calf. Father, remove from me the shortness of breath, heart palpitations, coughing, excessive sweating, dizziness, clammy and discolored skin (cyanosis) and fever. Holy Spirit, come. I thank You for energy and vitality, and I know that You are doing a miracle in my respiratory system even as I am praying this. You are protecting me from danger, and I will love long and live strong. "I will cause breath to enter you, and you shall live" (Ezekiel 37:5). In Jesus' name, Amen.

Tuberculosis (TB) Healing Prayer

Jesus, please heal my lungs from this infection of tuberculosis. I am in desperate need of Your touch so that not only can I be rid of TB myself, but also so that I might not be contagious to anyone else. Holy Spirit, come. Please heal me from the fever and chills, the loss of appetite and weight loss, the fatigue and night sweats, shortness of breath and chest pain, and the swollen lymph nodes and coughing up blood. Of course, I realize that my lymph nodes are swollen because they are attempting to drain off the infection as my immune system fights hard to heal it. Lord, I receive that healing! You have designed my body to fight for healing, and I declare that I shall have it. "Nor is he served by human hands, as though he needed anything, since he himself gives to all mankind life and breath and everything" (Acts 17:25). In Jesus' name, Amen.

Whooping Cough (Pertussis) Healing Prayer

Great Healer, touch my body and my entire respiratory system right now, healing me of this whooping cough. You alone have the power to put an end to this respiratory tract infection and the chronic, severe cough that accompanies it. Lord, heal me from the fever, fatigue, vomiting and inability to breathe. Also touch my nearby sinuses and heal me from the watery eyes, runny nose, sneezing and nasal congestion. Bring an utter end to the bacteria called Bordetella pertussis in my system, and heal me of any resulting complications from all the coughing, such as abdominal hernias, broken blood vessels in the skin or eyes, and bruised or cracked ribs. I also trust You, God, to protect those around me; please do not allow them to catch this. I declare that those I love are safe from this infection and that I am on my way to healing. Holy Spirit, come. "The Spirit of God has made me, and the breath of the Almighty gives me life" (Job 33:4). I ask it all in the name of Jesus, Amen.

17

Digestive System

Mouth, Esophagus, Stomach, Liver, Small Intestines

Declaration

I am ready to receive any needed healing for my digestive system and then do whatever it takes to walk in divine health. I know that God does not make me sick, and I ask Him right now to show me the root of my condition, whether it be physical, emotional or spiritual. I am ready to pray the prayer of faith, reverse the curse and unleash the blessing. By God's grace, I will watch my words, maintain my miracle or wait on God's perfect timing for healing. Amen!

Digestive System Blessing

Your digestive system is hungry for change! While the system's tract stretches from the mouth to the

Digestive System

anus, it actually begins with your palate, so I first release over you a desire for whole foods, and then the willpower to choose them. Digestive discipline! As you eat, your saliva and digestive juices will do their jobs and break down your food without overactivity, reflux or indigestion. Your throat and esophagus are free from choking or blockages and connect perfectly to your pharynx, delivering food to your stomach without delay or irritation. All twenty feet of your small intestines—the duodenum, jejunum and ileum—are working together with the enzymes created by your liver and pancreas to break down fat, protein and carbohydrates. Your liver is being supernaturally cleansed right now and will better purify your blood, while your gallbladder will produce adequate bile and help distribute the digesting food into your large intestine. All passageways are healthy and free from bloating, ulcers, nausea and gastrointestinal (GI) disorders. Let it be done according to your faith and in the mighty name of Jesus!

Visit lauraharrissmith.com/blessings for the video blessing.

Your Digestive System's A-list

Avoid dairy, wheat, sugar, fried food, chili peppers, corn, alcohol; *stress*

Add avocadoes, raspberries, apples with skin, almonds, flaxseeds, ACV

Allow probiotic, prebiotic, L-glutamine; vitamins A, B complex, C, D

Apply ginger, fennel, peppermint, clove, cardamom, patchouli oils

Anoint with oil daily and pray needed healing prayers and body system blessings

Ask your doctor or health care provider before making regimen changes

Your Digestive System's Favorite . . .

Breakfast: smoothie—1 banana, 1 lemon, ½ avocado, 1 ginger root, 1 tablespoon coconut oil, ½ cup almond milk, ½ cup ice, stevia to taste

Lunch: black beans with bone broth, carrots, celery, garlic, onion, cumin, cayenne; cauliflower rice

Dinner: yam fries with guacamole, sugar snap peas, roasted broccoli; salmon or organic chicken

Snack: raspberries, blueberries, bananas, kiwi, cantaloupe, carrots, 70–80 percent cocoa organic dark chocolate (Lily's brand, made with stevia)

Testimony

"We had eaten out and arrived home late. I started feeling as if there were a lead weight in the pit of my stomach, and I thought I was going to be sick. I began to feel weak and decided to head for bed. I woke up a little over an hour later, realizing I must have food poisoning or be coming down with a nasty virus. I rushed dizzily and very unsteady on my feet to the bathroom. I was having cold sweats and knew throwing up was imminent. I ended up sitting on the floor of my bathroom until I could make it to my prayer chair to find my copy of Pastor Laura's digestive system declaration and blessing. I just began to pray and speak that blessing over my body, and almost immediately I began to feel better. I never did throw up and slept peacefully the rest of the night. There is an anointing and power in these body system blessings and prayers that needs to be tapped into. Let the Lord minister to you as you pray these and receive your healing today!" ~Dawn

After reading the blessings and prayers, send all testimonies large and small to healing@lauraharrissmith.com.

Digestive System Healing Prayers

Celiac Disease Healing Prayer

Lord, I am ready to eat and not feel such discomfort. I am ready for food to be my friend and not my enemy. I am also ready for the foods we all eat to be less genetically modified so that they are less inflammatory to society. Until then (since that day may never come without major legislation changes), Holy Spirit, come. I need Your twofold help. I ask You to touch my body so that it is free from celiac disease. But I also ask You to point me to the right nutritious foods so that, through the elimination of heavily modified foods (such as wheat and gluten), I might be free of these symptoms forever. Remind me to adhere to this chapter's A-list advice. I thank You that through this I will not always have to put up with the gas, belching, diarrhea, cramping, fatty stools, bloating, nausea, abdominal pain, mouth ulcers, burning in the chest and indigestion. I also thank You for freedom from the more serious issues of anemia, bone loss, osteoporosis, joint pain, malnutrition and delayed puberty or slow growth. "And God said, 'Behold, I have given you every plant yielding seed that is on the face of all the earth, and every tree with seed in its fruit. You shall have them for food'" (Genesis 1:29). I thank You for this twofold healing, Lord. It's in Jesus' name I pray, Amen.

Cholestasis Healing Prayer

Jesus, I turn to You for relief from this severe pain in my upper right abdomen. I need You to heal this reduction or stoppage of bile flow in my body, and please touch my gallbladder, liver and pancreas to make that happen. Please take the bloating, cramping, itching, fatty stools, pale feces, dark urine and loss of appetite and remove them for good. Brighten my eyes and heal them of the yellow discoloration due to the accumulation of bilirubin (bile) that has escaped into my bloodstream. Energize me and give me a strategy for dietary changes, knowing that processed meats, bacon, hot dogs and dairy products are huge triggers for me. I will not be the cause of my own pain. It will not be said of me that I am among those "whose end is destruction, whose god is their appetite, and whose glory is in their shame, who set their minds on earthly things" (Philippians 3:18–19 NASB). Holy Spirit, come. Help me set my mind on health and healing. I ask it all in Your name, Amen.

Colic (for Babies) Healing Prayer

Note: All babies cry, but before self-diagnosing colic, make sure you check with your pediatrician and confirm that there is nothing medically wrong with your baby. Colic is defined as unexplained, inconsolable crying in a healthy infant for three or more hours a day, three or four days a week, for a period of time that lasts three or four weeks. Its incidence peaks at six weeks of age, and it usually ends by the time a baby is three or four months old.

Lord, I am worried about my baby's constant crying, which seems only to worsen at night when I am tired. We have fed, burped, diapered and rocked the baby, and nothing seems to be working. Holy Spirit, come. Bring Your peace to this little one and show me if there is something I can do in the natural to calm him or her. Since we have done everything we can do under the supervision of our doctor, I pray that You Yourself would ease our baby's extreme fussiness, screaming, discomfort, bodily tension and stiffened limbs and abdomen, as only You can do. Jesus, if we are dealing with childhood migraines, food allergies, an underdeveloped digestive system, overfeeding or underfeeding, or a bacterial imbalance in the tummy, please heal it right now in the name of Jesus. Finally, help us remember that babies are very sensitive to family stress or anxiety, so bring peace to our entire household. "Like newborn infants, long for the pure spiritual milk, that by it you may grow up into salvation" (1 Peter 2:2). In the name of Jesus, Amen.

Colon Polyps Healing Prayer

G od, after being told I have colon polyps, I am turning to You. I ask You to heal me of the small clumps of cells that have formed on the lining of my colon, whether they are nonneoplastic (including hyperplastic, inflammatory or hamartomatous polyps) or neoplastic (including adenomas and serrated types). I know that the neoplastic have a greater risk of becoming cancerous, as do the larger polyps, but I am turning that fear over to You and trading it in for healing. Put an end to the rectal bleeding, hemorrhoids and any resulting anemia from the blood loss. Return my stool color and bowel habits to normal and remove the pain from my gut. I declare that cancer is not in my future, and I accept Your wisdom on eating the right foods so that I might walk in divine health and stay ahead of the enemy, who is always wanting to steal, kill and destroy. "Or do you not know that your body is a temple of the Holy Spirit within you, whom you have from God? You are not your own, for you were bought with a price. So glorify God in your body" (1 Corinthians 6:19–20). Holy Spirit, come. I ask it all in Your name, Amen.

Constipation Healing Prayer

F ather, please help get my digestive and excretory systems moving and working together to help keep me regular. I need relief from the bloating, nausea, gas, constipation and belly cramping. And God, the pain can become unbearable, so I need You to heal whatever is wrong so that I am no longer experiencing that kind of intense pain. Holy Spirit, come. Help me abide by the advice on this chapter's A-list so that my body stays nourished and my bowel movements become regular. "And Jesus said to him, 'Go your way; your faith has made you well'" (Mark 10:52). In the name of Jesus I pray, Amen.

Eating Disorders Healing Prayer

Lord, I feel imprisoned by this issue that is part psychological and part physical, but since it is affecting my food and diet, I am going to begin by praying for my digestive tract and the choices I make concerning it. If it is anorexia nervosa, then heal me of my preoccupation with weight, the inability to maintain appropriate weight, and hiding my weight loss with layers. If it is bulimia nervosa, then heal me of all binging tendencies, along with the self-induced vomiting and resulting dental issues. If it is binge eating disorder, then put an end to my episodes of binge eating, the inability to stop eating and the resulting disgust with myself. If it is pica, then cure me of the desire to consume nonfood items like soap, chalk or string. If it is rumination disorder, then help me stop the consumption of regurgitated food. If it is ARFID (avoidant/restrictive food intake disorder), then help me not be so picky when I eat, or be fearful of choking or vomiting. Finally, if it is OSFED (other specified feeding or eating disorder), then heal me of the various symptoms, including binging on large amounts of food and then expressing the need to burn off all the calories I consumed. Holy Spirit, come. Heal my mind from all depression, anxiety and self-loathing [see those healing prayers in chapter 26]. My digestive tract is not only the source of all nourishment for my body, but also the seat of 70 percent of my immune system, so I know that through this healing comes health and protection for my whole body. "Beloved, I pray that all may go well with you and that you may be in good health, as it goes well with your soul" (3 John 2). In Jesus' name I pray all these things, Amen.

Esophagitis Healing Prayer

God, I need healing from this esophagitis. Deliver me from the chest pain, difficulty swallowing, heartburn, nausea, vomiting, belching and coughing. Help me not to fear eating, or abstain from eating due to fear of food getting stuck, and please remove the swelling from my esophagus. Holy Spirit, come. My immune system and digestive system are intertwined and need nourishing. So, Lord, help me keep them nourished with foods that are a blessing to them both. "And he humbled you and let you hunger and fed you with manna, which you did not know, nor did your fathers know, that he might make you know that man does not live by bread alone, but man lives by every word that comes from the mouth of the LORD" (Deuteronomy 8:3). I ask it all in Your name, Amen.

Food Poisoning Healing Prayer

Holy Spirit, come. I am in great pain. I believe I have come into contact with food contaminated by either a virus, bacteria, toxins or parasites. Please rid my body of these foreign invaders! I know the fever means my body is fighting, so strengthen my immune system to fight and win. Heal me of the abdominal and rectal pain, nausea, vomiting, diarrhea, bloating, gagging, stomach cramps and gas. Bring an end to the dizziness, chills, light-headedness, loss of appetite, weakness and sweating. And Lord, I know that I can rebuke dehydration or I can go drink a glass of water, so convince me of the importance of both. "Food is for the stomach and the stomach is for food, but God will do away with both of them. Yet the body is not for immorality, but for the Lord, and the Lord is for the body" (1 Corinthians 6:13 NASB). I pray all of this in Jesus' name, Amen.

> Note: Once your stomach is settled, consider my "B Well" recovery diet: bananas, berries, boiled eggs, brown rice or baked potato with butter. To drink: ginger tea or "Zevia" (stevia ginger ale).

Gallstones and Gallbladder Disease (Including Cholecystitis) Healing Prayer

Father, please deliver me from the pain of these gallstones. Heal me of the stones themselves and of the discomfort and cramping they bring. Give me freedom from the nausea, vomiting, indigestion, back pain and upper-right abdominal pain. Prevent any further digestive juices from hardening and forming these deposits, and prevent those stones present from blocking the tube leading to my small intestines (cholecystitis). I pray that the issues and symptoms will go, by Your command, and that surgery will not even be needed. Holy Spirit, come. I know that You will bless my entire digestive system and restore it. "Therefore I tell you, do not be anxious about your life, what you will eat or what you will drink, nor about your body, what you will put on. Is not life more than food, and the body more than clothing?" (Matthew 6:25). It is in the name of Jesus I pray, Amen.

Gastritis Healing Prayer

Lord, please heal me of this upper abdominal pain. I give You the symptoms and ask You to relieve them all—the nausea, vomiting, indigestion, belching, heartburn and loss of appetite. Remove the gnawing and burning ache in my upper belly, and any pain radiating to the back. Bring peace to my entire upper GI tract. Lord, if this came from infection, please cure it, and if from injury, then please heal that, too. If it was from taking too many over-the-counter pain relievers, then show me a new strategy to remove those from my regimen since they can cause so much intestinal damage. Order my life to remove unnecessary stress, which I know can wreak intestinal havoc on my body. Holy Spirit, come. Convict me to adhere to this chapter's A-list for optimum digestive system health. "Jesus said to them, 'I am the bread of life; whoever comes to me shall not hunger, and whoever believes in me shall never thirst'" (John 6:35). In the name of Jesus I pray all of this, Amen.

GERD (Acid Reflux) Healing Prayer

God, I am ready to eat and not hurt afterward. I am asking you to heal this GERD and the constant heartburn, nausea and regurgitation. Please take this bitter taste from my mouth, along with the dry cough and the upper abdominal discomfort. I am ready to lie down at night and not be in pain from my stomach acids or bile flowing into my food pipe and irritating the lining. Holy Spirit, come. Finally, help me steer clear of the unhealthy foods listed in this chapter's A-list that are not good for me and that are triggers, while gracing me to adhere to the A-list's best foods for me. "With the fruit of a man's mouth his stomach will be satisfied; He will be satisfied with the product of his lips" (Proverbs 18:20 NASB).

Hepatitis A, B, C, D, E Healing Prayer

Lord Jesus, hepatitis is a scary diagnosis, but I know You are with me and are carrying me through this battle. Regardless of my form of hepatitis, I need You to touch my liver and make it whole. Please take away all this abdominal pain, fatigue, loss of appetite, nausea, diarrhea, vomiting and itching. Please heal the joint paint, fever, chills, dark urine, yellowing of my eyes and skin (jaundice) and swollen blood vessels. I also ask You to keep me from the depression, weight loss and active liver failure. I know that You have healing in store for Me, because Your Word tells me so. I thank You right now for that promise. Holy Spirit, come. I declare that I will not eat things that will prevent the healing work You are doing in my body. And now, Lord, help me stick to this chapter's A-list advice for optimum digestive health. "So, whether you eat or drink, or whatever you do, do all to the glory of God" (1 Corinthians 10:31). In the name of Jesus I pray, Amen.

Hiatal Hernia Healing Prayer

Heavenly Father, I need Your healing touch in my digestive tract, especially where my esophagus connects to my stomach. Please cause my stomach no longer to bulge through the opening in my diaphragm and push up into my chest. Command everything to go back to its place, taking with it all the chest and abdominal discomfort. Thank You also for no more nausea, regurgitation, heartburn, throat irritation, belching and vomiting. Holy Spirit, come. I declare that I will eat without pain and digest without interference. "The righteous has enough to satisfy his appetite" (Proverbs 13:25 NASB). In Jesus' name I pray, Amen.

Inflammatory Bowel Disease (IBD, Crohn's, Ulcerative Colitis) Healing Prayer

Jesus, in Your name I am running to You for healing. I am weary from the abdominal pain, rectal bleeding, bowel obstructions, diarrhea, anal fissures, nausea, vomiting, gas and cramping. I am tired of feeling tired, anemic, weak, fevered and occasionally embarrassed and depressed at the lifestyle I am often forced to lead. I refuse to live my life dreading flare-ups and having my schedule not be my own due to the constant, looming potential of hospitalizations and a lifetime on immunosuppressants. I refuse to be unhealthy and be constantly trying to gain back weight to keep from looking frail. Holy Spirit, come. I know that You do not want me to be a hostage to my intestinal tract and its unpredictable demands, and I also know that You do not want my enemy to triumph over me. Heal me, O Great God, from the joint pain, too, for I am too young to feel this old. Finally, I come against the "fact" that this is a lifelong illness, that this will result in surgery, and that I have a high risk for colorectal cancer. I know the facts, but I also know the truth, which is that You are my Healer. So I command the facts to submit themselves to the truth right now. God, I am going to change how I eat and take responsibility for my part in this, abiding by this chapter's A-list advice and cooperating with You for healing by abstaining from foods that undo the brand-new health You are giving me. "For anyone who eats and drinks without discerning the body eats and drinks judgment on himself. That is why many of you are weak and ill, and some have died" (1 Corinthians 11:29–30). I ask all of this in Your name, Jesus. Amen.

Irritable Bowel Syndrome (IBS) Healing Prayer

Father in heaven, You are my Great Physician and I need You to do what no doctor can do: Heal me of IBS. Only You know how weary I am of the nausea, cramping and discomfort, not to mention the inconvenient bowel changes I have experienced, such as the constipation, diarrhea, gas, indigestion and the inability to empty my bowel. Lord, it is all so depressing, so I ask You also to heal me of the depression and anxiety that I often fight off. Holy Spirit, come. Heal my body, mind and appetite. Give me a desire for this chapter's A-list foods that will keep my gut healthy, for I know that is what You want. I declare to You today that I will cooperate with You and not ingest that which can undo the digestive miracle You are giving me. "Blessed are those who hunger and thirst for righteousness, for they shall be satisfied" (Matthew 5:6), to which I say yes and amen. In Jesus' name I pray, Amen.

Jaundice Healing Prayer

Note: As a matter of testimony, in 1990 my newborn son developed severe jaundice that lingered for about two months, despite our hospital's best efforts to cure him. Finally, after being told his little liver was in grave danger, a total blood transfusion was ordered, but in the early nineties the first big scares with HIV-infected blood donors had surfaced, and we were apprehensive. Some friends suggested we have Jhason prayed over for healing—something we had never had to do before—and we stepped out in faith and did it the weekend before the transfusion. When we took him to the hospital on Monday morning, his blood was clean, and his body and liver were totally healed. We have never doubted God's healing power since! I will recount for you the prayer we prayed (which can be used on anyone of any age), but remember that it is not just the words on the page, but the faith in your heart and even the desperation in your spirit that God will visit.

Jesus, I come to you right now and ask You to heal _____'s body, particularly the liver. I ask You to take away the jaundice and unclog any obstructions of the bile ducts that are causing excessive amounts of the yellow pigment bilirubin to accumulate and discolor his or her eyes and skin. Holy Spirit, come. Cleanse the liver and blood so that they might do their jobs better and lower the bilirubin level promptly. "The LORD protects him and keeps him alive . . . you do not give him up to the will of his enemies. The LORD sustains him on his sickbed; in his illness you restore him to full health" (Psalm 41:2–3). In Jesus' name I pray, Amen.

Leaky Gut Syndrome (Intestinal Permeability) Healing Prayer

Lord, the lining of my stomach has been compromised. The epithelial cells that are normally linked by tight junction proteins have malfunctioned and are no longer protecting and controlling what passes between my intestinal lining and bloodstream. God, as I implement this chapter's A-list, repair my body and obliterate these symptoms of diarrhea, rectal bleeding, gastric ulcers, fatigue, celiac disease, allergies, autoimmune diseases, irritable bowel syndrome, malnutrition, psoriasis or other skin inflammations, thyroid issues, hair loss and of course the mood swings and depression tendencies. Knowing that 70 percent of my immune system is in my gut, heal me there so my entire being might be better protected against future sickness. Holy Spirit, come. I receive Your invitation to make the changes necessary for better health, adhering to this chapter's A-list nutritional advice. "Behold, I stand at the door and knock. If anyone hears my voice and opens the door, I will come in to him and eat with him, and he with me" (Revelation 3:20). It's in the name of Jesus I pray, Amen.

Liver Disease / Cirrhosis Healing Prayer

Jesus, I lay this overwhelming diagnosis of cirrhosis at Your feet. Experts say that the liver damage caused by cirrhosis cannot be reversed, but I know that all things are possible with You. Please relieve me of the abdominal pain, excess abdominal fluid, rectal bleeding, loss of appetite, nausea, vomiting blood, gas, water retention and weight gain or loss. I am tired of being tired. I am weary from the mental confusion and ask You to touch my mind. Please remove all jaundice from me as You steady my bilirubin levels to accomplish this. Thank You for healing me from all bruising—bodily and in my blood vessels—and the enlarged veins around my abdomen. I declare that I will be hormonally balanced and will not have reduced hormone production, enlarged breasts, or swelling in my extremities, esophagus or elsewhere. Holy Spirit, come. Please do all these things without a liver transplant. But should You choose a surgical route to save my life, please guide me through the process physically and financially. First, however, I vow to You to receive Your wisdom on making necessary changes, especially if this diagnosis came because of alcohol overconsumption. "Wine is a mocker, strong drink a brawler, and whoever is led astray by it is not wise" (Proverbs 20:1). Also convict me and remind me to adhere to this chapter's A-list advice. I pray it all in Your name, Jesus. Amen.

Nausea/Vomiting Healing Prayer

Lord, right now I call for an end to this nausea. If there is a substance in my body that needs to exit and not be digested, then Lord, let it come up and out quickly [see the food poisoning prayer in this chapter]. But, God, if this is just a queasy interruption to my day, please calm my digestive system and bring peace to my whole body. Holy Spirit, come. If I have eaten something that does not agree with me, may I be wise enough to listen to my body and never eat it again, realizing that everything I put into my mouth affects my entire being during its journey through my body. And if this nausea is caused due to anxiety and fear, please remove it and help me put my faith in You. "Do you not understand that everything that goes into the mouth passes into the stomach, and is eliminated?" (Matthew 15:17 NASB). In Jesus' name I pray, Amen.

Ulcers Healing Prayer

Father, first help me determine how I became vulnerable to these ulcers in my body. If it be genetics, I declare that I am Your child and therefore not an heir to anything but good health. If it be stress, then please help me eliminate all negativity and obvious stress triggers in my life. And if I am around people whom I cannot distance myself from entirely—such as family— then please give me the grace to stay and be at peace as You work on my behalf. Take these symptoms right now, Lord, of the chest pain, indigestion, heartburn, gas, nausea, upper abdominal discomfort, vomiting, fatigue and rectal bleeding (brown blood that has been digested, having gone from the upper GI tract through the digestion process). Holy Spirit, come. Teach me to nourish my digestive system with this chapter's A-list foods, knowing that You love it when I use the things You have created to enable me to walk in divine health. Help me find freedom from food choices that are harming me. "For such men are slaves, not of our Lord Christ but of their own appetites" (Romans 16:18 NASB). In the name of Jesus, Amen.

18

Excretory System

Large Intestines, Colon, Rectum

Declaration

I am ready to receive any needed healing for my excretory system and then do whatever it takes to walk in divine health. I know that God does not make me sick, and I ask Him right now to show me the root of my condition, whether it be physical, emotional or spiritual. I am ready to pray the prayer of faith, reverse the curse and unleash the blessing. By God's grace, I will watch my words, maintain my miracle or wait on God's perfect timing for healing. Amen!

Excretory System Blessing

As your upper GI tract delivers your healthy foods farther down the food chain to your large intestines—that five or six feet of muscular tubing called the colon— your lower bowel will receive the foods and properly

Excretory System

absorb their nutrients for optimum health throughout your entire body. Beginning with the opening to the large intestines (the cecum), and then traveling on to the ascending (right) colon, the transverse (across) colon, and the descending (left) colon, all valves function perfectly, and each part of your colon is free from ulcerative tendencies and any bowel diseases. Your sigmoid colon connects perfectly to your rectum for proper elimination by the anus, and you will enjoy perfect digestion and regularity. I release that blessing to you right now. Let it be done according to your faith and in the mighty name of Jesus!

Visit lauraharrissmith.com/blessings for the video blessing.

Your Excretory System's A-list

Avoid caffeine, red meat, white rice, dairy, wheat, chips, fast food, alcohol

Add 8 glasses water daily (or 4 to 5 glasses with a 50 percent raw produce diet), legumes, nuts; *saunas*

Allow probiotics, magnesium taurate; vitamins B complex, C; 1 tablespoon daily coconut oil

Apply cinnamon, lavender, fennel ginger, spearmint, peppermint, lemon oils

Anoint with oil daily and pray needed healing prayers and body system blessings

Ask your doctor or health care provider before making regimen changes

Your Excretory System's Favorite . . .

Breakfast: steel-cut oatmeal with stevia or Swerve; blueberries, rhubarb, walnuts, coffee (decaf)

Lunch: cauliflower rice and black beans with onion, cumin, turmeric, cayenne and guacamole

Dinner: stir-fry with broccoli, cabbage, bok choy, gluten-free soy sauce; cauliflower rice; arugula/kale salad.

Snack: figs, prunes, pears, kiwi, apples, raspberries, roasted chickpeas (toss 1 drained can with olive oil, chili powder, pink salt and roast at 350° for 30 minutes)

Testimony

"I have been praying Laura's 15 body system blessings over myself, and last week I was having daily symptoms of diverticulitis—a dull ache in my left side. I continued to pray the excretory system blessing over myself, and I also massaged lavender and cinnamon oil on that area and on my lower abdomen one night before bed. Next day—gone and has not returned! After having diverticulitis SO many times, it's awesome there was no need for a human doctor!" ~Fay

After reading the blessings and prayers, send all testimonies large and small to healing@lauraharrissmith.com.

Excretory System Healing Prayers

Anal Fissure Healing Prayer

God, You have created my body to eliminate the foods I eat, and I would prefer to do that without pain! Please heal the small rectal tear(s) that occurred when I was pushing or straining, and also put an end to any bleeding or cracked skin surrounding the fissure. I thank You for pain-free bowel movements and that this important process will not be disrupted in my daily routine. Holy Spirit, come. "But for you who fear my name, the sun of righteousness shall rise with healing in its wings. You shall go out leaping like calves from the stall" (Malachi 4:2). In Jesus' name I believe and receive, Amen.

Anorectal Abscess (Perianal Abscess) Healing Prayer

Jesus, I ask You for relief right now, in Your name. Please heal my entire excretory system, especially the portions that are swollen, tender, itching and abscessed. Father, heal any infection and resulting fever, pus or discharge. And, Lord, if this wound is the result of a sexually transmitted disease, please bring healing to my spirit first, and then to my mind and body. If this is the result of a digestive disorder, then touch my digestive and excretory systems and bring them both into perfect harmony. "'He himself bore our sins' in his body on the cross, so that we might die to sins and live for righteousness; 'by his wounds you have been healed'" (1 Peter 2:24 NIV). Holy Spirit, come. In Your name I pray, Amen.

Bowel Incontinence Healing Prayer

Lord, I am tired of this embarrassing issue, and I ask You to heal my body so that it functions as You created it to. Help me with every urge and its timing, and whether this issue is due to age or due to giving birth, I ask You to heal my excretory system so that it functions when it needs to function, and not until then.

209

Holy Spirit, come. Mend any accompanying problems of pain, diarrhea, gas, bloating and constipation. If there is an underlying intestinal issue, please touch my digestive system and bring healing and strength there, too. "So do not fear, for I am with you; do not be dismayed, for I am your God. I will strengthen you and help you; I will uphold you with my righteous right hand" (Isaiah 41:10 NIV). I pray these things in the name of Jesus, Amen.

Diarrhea Healing Prayer

Lord Jesus, my digestive tract seems inflamed, as evidenced by the fact that my excretory system is not producing anything solid. Would You please touch both systems right now and bring balance and healing to them? Please provide me relief from the loose and watery stools, abdominal pain and cramping, nausea, bloating and even any fever or rectal bleeding. Holy Spirit, come. As I nourish my body with the right foods from this chapter's A-list, add Your "super" to my "natural" and bring supernatural healing and regularity, preventing any dehydration from occurring. May I remember to eat and drink as if my life depends on it, because it does! "Worship the LORD your God, and his blessing will be on your food and water. I will take away sickness from among you" (Exodus 23:25 NIV). In Jesus' name I pray it all, Amen.

Diverticulitis Healing Prayer

Heavenly Father, I come to You for healing in my digestive system, particularly my colon. Small, bulging pouches—diverticula—have been lining my digestive tract and causing me great pain whenever they are infected or inflamed. Please take from me the nausea, vomiting, intestinal tenderness, cramping, bloating, loss of appetite, chills and fever. I also ask You to heal me of the bowel changes, rectal bleeding, gas and constipation. Holy Spirit, come. Remind me to get enough rest, vegetable fiber and liquids. Bolster my appetite again and bless my efforts as I adhere to this chapter's A-list advice and fortify my entire excretory system. "Bless the LORD, O my soul, and all that is within me, bless his holy name! Bless the LORD, O my soul, and forget not all his benefits, who forgives all your iniquity, who heals all your diseases, who redeems your life from the pit, who crowns you with steadfast love and mercy, who satisfies you with good so that your youth is renewed like the eagle's" (Psalm 103:1–5). In the name of Jesus I pray, Amen.

Fecal Impaction (Blocked Bowel) Healing Prayer

Heavenly Father, this constipation has become an impaction, and the pain is almost too great to bear. Please get my excretory system moving again and make me regular, employing, of course, the help of my digestive system. Relieve me of the painful symptoms such as belly cramping, bloating, stool leakage, nausea, gas and the obstructions large or small. Holy Spirit, come. Whether the blockage is in the rectum, colon or even my upper GI tract, please remove it and put an end to the chronic constipation. "Then your light will break forth like the dawn, and your healing will quickly appear; then your righteousness will go before you, and the glory of the LORD will be your rear guard" (Isaiah 58:8 NIV). I ask it all in Your name, Lord. Amen.

Hemorrhoids (Piles) Healing Prayer

Lord, it would be a great blessing to be able to sit without discomfort and to experience pain-free elimination. I pray for healing in my body's rectal walls, and I ask that You would strengthen them and reduce the inflammation that has caused these piles to form. Whether internal or external, please take away the bleeding, swelling, itching and, most importantly, the pain and discomfort. Please protect me from any thrombosed hemorrhoids, where dangerous blood clots could add to the complications.

Holy Spirit, come. Get my digestive and excretory systems flowing smoothly, so that there is no longer the need for pushing and straining. "There is a time for everything . . . a time to heal" (Ecclesiastes 3:1–3 NIV). In Jesus' name, Amen.

Rectal Bleeding (Rectorrhagia) Healing Prayer

Jesus, I need You to heal my body from this alarming bleeding. There is obviously something wrong in my digestive and excretory systems, but I am calmed by the fact that You know what it is. Holy Spirit, come. Bring healing to my digestive tract [see the IBD and IBS healing prayers in chapter 17], or if the issue is more minor and just involves the rectal walls, please bring healing there, too [see the anal fissure prayer in this chapter]. If the bleeding is bright red, then I know that means it is "new blood" and there is an issue in my lower GI tract or colon. If the blood is brown or tarry, then that means it is "old blood" from higher up in the GI tract. Either way, You are my Healer, and I know You will restore me. Give me the desire and discipline to adhere to this chapter's A-list for a totally healthy excretory system, start to finish. "Lord, your discipline is good, for it leads to life and health. You restore my health and allow me to live" (Isaiah 38:16 NLT). In the name of Jesus I pray, Amen.

Rectal Prolapse Healing Prayer

God, I am turning to You for healing in my excretory system. Whether this rectal prolapse is the result of a weak anal wall, an anal injury, a misuse of the anal cavity or just multiple births by vaginal delivery, please touch my body at this time and bring the healing that only You can provide. Holy Spirit, come. Thank You in advance for deliverance from the protrusions, discharge, itchiness and constipation. I receive Your healing and the ability to eliminate without pain and to control bowel movements without incident. "He sent out his word and healed them, and delivered them from their destruction" (Psalm 107:20). I ask it all in Your name, Lord. Amen.

Rectovaginal Fistula Healing Prayer

Lord, I am in pain and need Your healing power. Please correct the improper connection between the lower portion of my large intestines—the rectum—and my vaginal wall. Whether the condition occurred as a result of childbirth, an inflammatory bowel disease or during pelvic radiation or surgery, I know that You can heal it perfectly. Holy Spirit, come. Please bring me relief from the pain, discharge, urinary tract infections (UTIs), gas and irritation. I also give You my stress over this condition—especially as it pertains to intimacy—and I know that You will take care of me. "'May they have abundant peace, both near and far,' says the Lord, who heals them" (Isaiah 57:19 NLT). Thank You, Jesus, and it is in Your name I pray all of this. Amen.

19

Urinary System
Kidneys, Bladder, Gallbladder

Declaration

I am ready to receive any needed healing for my urinary system and then do whatever it takes to walk in divine health. I know that God does not make me sick, and I ask Him right now to show me the root of my condition, whether it be physical, emotional or spiritual. I am ready to pray the prayer of faith, reverse the curse and unleash the blessing. By God's grace, I will watch my words, maintain my miracle or wait on God's perfect timing for healing. Amen!

Urinary System Blessing

Your urinary tract's ability to remove toxins from your body is its premier job, so I speak perfect harmony between its many parts so it can accomplish that and keep your entire body clean. Beginning with your kidneys

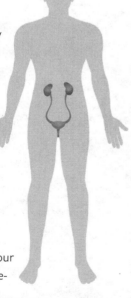

Urinary System

just below your rib cage—which work around the clock and produce between one and two quarts of urine a day—I speak a blessing of productivity and flow from the ureters down into the bladder. While you have no control of kidney function or the signals the bladder sends to the brain to tell you it is full, you do control bladder emptying (through the urethra and its sphincters) so I declare that you will have a healthy stream without leakage, blockage or infection. Total health and functionality to your entire urinary system, and healing from anything that prevents them! Let it be done according to your faith and in the mighty name of Jesus!

Visit lauraharrissmith.com/blessings for the video blessing.

Your Urinary System's A-list

Avoid excess protein and salt, sugar or honey, caffeine, dairy, licorice root

Add 8 glasses water (or 4 to 5 glasses with a 50 percent raw produce diet), cranberries, citrus; *walking*

Allow D-mannose, saw palmetto, probiotics; vitamins B6, C; magnesium taurate

Apply oregano, frankincense, myrrh, lemongrass, bergamot, clove oils

Anoint with oil daily and pray needed healing prayers and body system blessings

Ask your doctor or health care provider before making regimen changes

Your Urinary System's Favorite . . .

Breakfast: egg omelet with spinach, shitake mushroom, tomato; grapefruit; macadamia nuts

Lunch: buckwheat noodle (it is not wheat) stir-fried with mushroom, spinach, olive oil, garlic, bone broth

Dinner: arugula salad with bell peppers, celery, chicken with olive oil, parsley, garlic, dried cranberries

Snack: watermelon with mint, oranges, lemons, blueberries, strawberries, red grapes, macadamia nuts, pineapple, dandelion tea, green tea

Testimony

"I was experiencing great discomfort with a urinary tract infection and could not even sit due to the burning pain. I was at a friend's house watching a movie and was just pacing around trying to keep moving through the pain when my host finally noticed and offered me Laura's UTI home remedy concoction [see pages 221–222]. Within thirty minutes I could sit and in another thirty minutes my pain was gone. It is unheard of to find relief so fast with a UTI. It was explained to me that the remedy wouldn't cure the infection but that it would neutralize the uric acid and relieve the pain, giving some other remedies for the infection itself time to work. I was able to finish the movie and enjoy my evening, and then I drank another cup once home so I could sleep pain-free." ~Leo

After reading the blessings and prayers, send all testimonies large and small to healing@lauraharrissmith.com.

Urinary System Healing Prayers

Bladder Prolapse (Cystocele, Bladder Hernia) Healing Prayer

Lord, I am in need of healing in my urinary system, specifically my bladder. Please rebuild the supportive tissue between there and the vaginal wall that has stretched and prolapsed, and remove the pressure that has resulted from that injury. Whether it came after childbirth(s), heavy lifting, severe coughing or just muscle strains within the pelvic area, I know You can heal it. I pray that I can be free of the discomfort, frequent urges to urinate, leakage and reduced urine retention. Holy Spirit, come. I thank You in advance that I will be able to feel I have emptied my bladder when I urinate, and that my days of pelvic pressure will be gone. "And he said to her, 'Daughter, your faith has made you well; go in peace, and be healed of your disease'" (Mark 5:34). In Jesus' name I pray, Amen.

Chronic Kidney Disease (CKD) / Kidney Failure Healing Prayer

Father, after the blood test led to this diagnosis of CKD, perhaps the first thing I need to ask for healing from is the fear and dread that is trying to overtake my mind. I do not want to be bound to a lifetime of dialysis treatments in order to avoid renal failure. I thank You that treatments are available, but ultimately, I need a new set of kidneys, and I know You are able to provide that! Holy Spirit, come. Please revive my kidneys so that they once again filter waste and excess fluid that my body does not need. Take from me these symptoms of insufficient urine production, insomnia, swelling, nausea, fatigue, appetite loss, kidney damage, high blood pressure, chest pain, confusion, abnormal heart rhythm and the severe weight loss and sometimes gain that is associated with CKD. Restore my electrolyte levels so that balance comes to my entire body. If You choose a progressive remedy for me, such as a kidney transplant, then I accept Your will, Lord. But I remind You that miracles are free, and I know that You still are in the miracle-working business. Be glorified, Lord! "The LORD will sustain him upon his sickbed; in his illness, You restore him to health" (Psalm 41:3 NASB). In the name of Jesus I pray this, Amen.

Hematuria (Blood in Urine) Healing Prayer

God, the discoloration in my urine is alarming, but I trust that You are guiding me toward healing. If this is occurring due to a urinary tract infection (UTI), pyelonephritis/kidney infections, CKD, prostatitis/enlarged prostate, or kidney stones, then please heal these underlying conditions [see the healing prayers for all of these in this chapter]. But if it is being caused by strenuous exercise, cancer, medications or even an inherited disorder, please show us the root of the problem and bring Your healing there, too. Thank You in advance for removing the red blood cells from my urine, along with any blood clots or pain. "And the power of the Lord was with him to heal" (Luke 5:17). Holy Spirit, come. In Your name, I pray, Amen.

Incontinence Healing Prayer

Lord, I am asking for Your healing from this embarrassing problem of urinary incontinence. If it is stress incontinence, please strengthen the necessary muscles when I am laughing, coughing, sneezing or lifting. If it is urge incontinence, heal any underlying infection or any more severe condition such as diabetes. If it is overflow incontinence, then please cause my bladder to empty completely so that there is no more constant dribbling. If it is functional incontinence, please heal the physical or mental impairment that is keeping me from making it to the toilet in time. Holy Spirit, come. Thank You for healing my urinary tract muscles for optimum bladder control. "Rise and go your way; your faith has made you well" (Luke 17:19). In Jesus' name, Amen.

Interstitial Cystitis (Painful Bladder Syndrome) Healing Prayer

Jesus, it seems that my nervous system and urinary system are not communicating well with one another, and signals are getting disrupted between my bladder and brain. I know that there is no infection and that this is not a UTI, but the pain is real, and I am asking You to remove it. Lord, please also take from me the pelvic pressure, frequent urges to urinate, bladder spasms and any pain during intercourse. Heal any bleeding, scarring and inflammation to the wall of the bladder, too. I am ready for my nights to be restful and pain free, and for my quality of life during the day to be better. Holy Spirit, come. Thank You for hearing my prayer. "Our bodies are buried in brokenness, but they will be raised in glory. They are buried in weakness, but they will be raised in strength" (1 Corinthians 15:43 NLT). In the mighty name of Jesus, Amen.

Kidney Infection (Pyelonephritis) Healing Prayer

Heavenly Father, please remove this infection from my body that seems to have started in my urethra or bladder and traveled to my kidneys. Take with it the pelvic inflammation, back pain, groin discomfort and abdominal or flank pain. In the mighty, healing name of Jesus I command every symptom to go, including the fever, chills, back pain, cloudy or bloody urine, foul-smelling urine, frequent urination and those pesky UTIs. Increase my appetite again so that I might be less fatigued and so my body can continue to fight off the infection. "God anointed Jesus of Nazareth with the Holy Spirit and with power. He went about doing good and healing all who were oppressed by the devil, for God was with him" (Acts 10:38). Holy Spirit, come. I ask this all in Jesus' name, Amen.

Kidney Stones Healing Prayer

Lord, I am desperate for You to help relieve this pain in my urinary system—the pain in my back, the pain in my side and the pain when I urinate. Please dissolve the hard mineral and acid salt deposits that have stuck together and formed in my concentrated urine, and may each stone's residue leave my body without major discomfort. As the residue exits, I thank You in advance for relief from the nausea, vomiting, sweating and blood in my urine. May I have the discipline to abide by this chapter's A-list for foods that will nourish and not harm my urinary system. "Have I not commanded you? Be strong and courageous. Do not be frightened, and do not be dismayed, for the LORD your God is with you wherever you go" (Joshua 1:9). Holy Spirit, come. In Jesus' name, Amen.

Overactive Bladder (OAB) Healing Prayer

Lord Jesus, I am weary of feeling as though my bladder is controlling my social life and choices. Please reveal what the root cause of this issue is (possible enlarged prostate [men]; possibly due to childbirth or pregnancy [women]; possible diabetes [both genders], etc.). Lord, it is embarrassing and uncomfortable, so I ask You to remove every symptom, including the bladder spasms, leakage, frequent urges to urinate and even bedwetting. I am also looking very forward to not having to use the bathroom so much during the night, which will lead to greater rest and improved overall health for me. "Heal the sick . . . and say to them, 'The kingdom of God has come near to you'" (Luke 10:9). Holy Spirit, come. In Jesus' name I pray in faith, Amen.

Prostatitis (Enlarged Prostate) Healing Prayer

Heavenly Father, I humbly ask You to heal my body of this inconvenient and sometimes painful disorder in my urinary system. Remove from me every symptom, including the difficulty urinating, frequent urination at night, lack of urinary retention, and blood in my urine. I thank You in advance for no more flu symptoms, chills, fever and fatigue (in severe cases). In Your name, I also command all the pain and inflammation to go, whether it be pain in my groin, pelvis, genitals, bladder, lower abdomen, prostate or even any rectal discomfort. I surrender to You my fear of prostate cancer, and I know that You will give me wisdom on how to proceed. Holy Spirit, come. You are my Healer, and I know You have only my good in mind. Grace me to nourish my urinary system with the foods on this chapter's A-list, so that I might not work against Your healing plan for me. "And he went throughout all Galilee, teaching in their synagogues and proclaiming the gospel of the kingdom and healing every disease and every affliction among the people" (Matthew 4:23). I ask it all in Your healing name, Jesus. Amen.

Urinary Tract Infection (UTI) Healing Prayer

Jesus, please remove this painful burning in my urinary tract and bring healing to my entire urinary system. Bring relief to every part of it, Lord, including my urethra, bladder and even my kidneys. Thank You for removing the pain and cramping from my pelvis, bladder, back, abdomen and groin. And by Your authority I command all other symptoms to go, such as the painful urination, frequent urination, blood in my urine, cloudy or dark urine, genital irritation, nausea, vomiting and fever. I would rather You do this instead of my having to take antibiotics that would kill the good flora in my gut, which is where 70 percent of my immune system is. Antibiotics leave me vulnerable to illness because sometimes it can take six months to rebuild the good flora. Holy Spirit, come. You are my Healer, so I wait on You. "And this is the confidence that we have toward him, that if we ask anything according to his will He hears us" (1 John 5:14). In Your healing name I pray, Amen.

Note: Quick pain relief tip for UTIs: (1) Fill a tall glass halfway with water and add 1 heaping teaspoon of baking soda and 2 tablespoons of apple cider vinegar (make sure the ACV you use has the organic "mother root" and is cloudy looking). Drink entirely once the bubbles settle down, or drink the water and soda alone and then take the ACV by spoon to avoid the bubble reaction. (2) Go to the bathroom after half an hour. (3) Immediately mix another glass of the same ingredients, and once the bubbles settle down a bit, drink it again all at once. Over the next half hour, you should begin to feel relief from the pain. You can do this again if necessary, and can do it a couple of times a day while you are dealing with the infection itself. This does not cure the UTI, but it neutralizes the uric acid in the urine and brings the body to a more alkaline place, which often eliminates the pain entirely. To deal with the infection itself, drink 100 percent cranberry juice constantly. Dilute 50/50 with water if necessary, or just take D-mannose in tablet or powder form (the main ingredient in cranberry juice). Finally, every 3 hours drink 3 drops in water of medicinal grade oil of oregano, which is nature's antibiotic.

20

Reproductive System
Ovaries, Testes

Declaration

I am ready to receive any needed healing for my reproductive system and hormones and then do whatever it takes to walk in divine health. I know that God does not make me sick, and I ask Him right now to show me the root of my condition, whether it be physical, emotional or spiritual. I am ready to pray the prayer of faith, reverse the curse and unleash the blessing. By God's grace, I will watch my words, maintain my miracle or wait on God's perfect timing for healing. Amen!

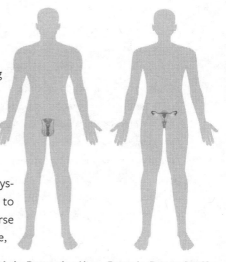

Male Reproductive System   Female Reproductive System

Reproductive System Blessing for Women

God's provision for life and legacy rests in your reproductive system. I release total health over your entire system, for the organs themselves and the hormones that flow to them. If you desire motherhood, I speak a blessing over your ovaries so you will have the perfect hormonal balance for egg production, perfect deliverance of the ova for fertilization, perfect conception in the fallopian tubes and complete plantation in the uterus, which all result in a healthy child. If you are not seeking motherhood at present, I call your body blessed with perfect hormonal balance that results in optimum gynecological health. Whichever group you are in, I declare "the curse" is broken off you for painful monthly cycles [see the painful menstrual periods healing prayer ahead, if this is you]. Finally, I speak grace for celibacy if you are not married and are experiencing the blessing of being fully devoted to the Lord in His service. Let it be done according to your faith and in the mighty name of Jesus!

Reproductive System Blessing for Men

God's provision for life and legacy rests in your reproductive system. I release total health over your entire system, for the organs themselves and the hormones that flow to them. If you desire fatherhood, I speak the blessing of God over your ability to produce, maintain and transport male reproductive cells (sperm) and over your body's ability to deliver those in its protective carrier fluid (semen). And I speak grace for celibacy if you are not married and are experiencing the blessing of being fully devoted to the Lord in His service. I speak youthfulness and hormonal vitality (through testosterone) into your body to fulfill the calling of God on your life with energy, whether it be as His servant or as a husband and father (or both). Let it be done according to your faith and in the mighty name of Jesus!

Visit lauraharrissmith.com/blessings for the video blessings.

Your Reproductive System's A-list

Avoid alcohol, sugar, PFC (in nonstick pans), BPA plastic, pesticides; *stress*

Add leafy greens, leafy greens, leafy greens, leafy greens, leafy greens!

Allow fish oil, folic acid; vitamins A, B complex, D3; magnesium taurate, calcium

Apply clary sage, ginger, yarrow, geranium, fennel, rose, ylang-ylang oils

Anoint with oil daily and pray needed healing prayers and body system blessings

Ask your doctor or health care provider before making regimen changes

Your Reproductive System's Favorite . . .

Breakfast: stewed apples with cinnamon, butter, pecans, stevia; avocado with cayenne; nut butters

Lunch: yam fries with guacamole; black bean soup with kale, bone broth, cumin, turmeric, chilies

Dinner: sweet potato with butter, coconut oil, cinnamon; leafy green salad with almonds; lean chicken

Snack: 70–80 percent cocoa organic dark chocolate, peaches, figs, plums, sunflower seeds, almonds, pecans, walnuts, watermelon, roasted kale chips, tea made with orange peel shavings

Testimony

"I have been praying Laura's 15 body system blessings over myself. The first thing I noticed when I was praying them was a sense of God's peace and presence. I printed off each one and taped them to my wall. I had been praying them all, but sometimes I would just focus on certain body systems. A few days ago, I started my monthly cycle. I've always had painful ones. Lots of cramps, nausea, vomiting and excessive bleeding, where double protection didn't even help. Lots of pain medication, heating pads and staying in bed. The next month, I would always have an overproduction of mucus. I had gone to the OB/GYN and was written a prescription, which I tried but wasn't comfortable on (and I'm a registered nurse). I prayed about it and didn't want those chemicals in my body. After praying about my symptoms, I started to notice them slowly getting better. I then started praying Laura's reproductive system blessing over myself. One day, I woke up and realized I had started my period and was beginning to get that yucky feeling. I immediately got up and sat on the edge of my bed, looking at all the prayer blessings on my wall. I prayed out loud the reproductive blessing one time, and then all my symptoms went away, and I haven't had any trouble since!" ~Jean

After reading the blessings and prayers, send all testimonies large and small to healing@lauraharrissmith.com.

Reproductive System Healing Prayers

Endometriosis Healing Prayer

Note: I was born to a mother who suffered greatly with endometriosis. After seven years of pain, and even after she underwent half a hysterectomy (an oophorectomy, which is the removal of one ovary and one fallopian tube), I was finally conceived. Never give up!

Jesus, I am ready to be free from the pain associated with endometriosis. Heal my body of this disorder that is making my endometrial tissue grow outside my uterus, in other places like my ovaries, fallopian tubes and pelvic region. Lord, may it stop thickening and bleeding during each cycle and becoming trapped in these foreign places, causing irritation, adhesions, scar tissue and even potentially causing my reproductive organs to stick to one another. Holy Spirit, come. Heal me of every symptom, including the heavy, painful or irregular menstruation and spotting. Please remove the constipation, nausea and abdominal fullness. And as for the pain, please deliver me from the cramping in my back, lower abdomen, pelvis, rectum, vagina and just the overall misery that comes with this disorder, Lord. I also do not want to lose my ability to bear children, so I declare that any children that I am to have, I will have! I resist infertility in the name of Jesus and trust Him to heal me. "There was a woman who had had a disabling spirit for eighteen years. She was bent over and could not fully straighten herself. When Jesus saw her, he called her over and said to her, 'Woman, you are freed from your disability.' And he laid his hands on her, and immediately she was made straight, and she glorified God" (Luke 13:11–13). In Jesus' name I believe and receive, Amen.

Infertility Healing Prayer

Lord, we want a baby [or another baby]. Our friends have children, our family members have children, and we want children, too [or more children]. Children are Your idea, and You tell us in the Bible to "be fruitful and multiply" (Genesis 1:28). So we know that it is Your will for us to ask for this child. Holy Spirit, come. Search our bodies and heal anything You find that is not right. Whether the issue be age, hormonal imbalances, low sperm count or medical treatments that are causing infertility, please heal us both. We receive Your blessing over every phase of conception—from ovulation to fertilization to implantation—and we will both make efforts to get healthier by following the A-list advice in this chapter. "You shall be blessed above all peoples. There shall not be male or female barren among you or among your livestock" (Deuteronomy 7:14). We thank You in advance for our new children, in the name of Jesus, Amen.

Low Testosterone (Low-T) Healing Prayer

God, I am ready to have my manhood restored. Please balance my hormones and cause my testosterone levels to rise to a healthy level, in Jesus' name. I need it for strong bones and muscles, but I also need it to be able to sleep well, maintain a proper weight and not experience sexual dysfunction. If there is an underlying condition that has robbed my body's testosterone—like diabetes, obesity or an infection—please heal that first, or show me a strategy for how to walk in Your divine health using the foods and strategies on this chapter's A-list. Holy Spirit, come. I trust You with my life, so of course I trust You with my manhood. "My son, be attentive to my words; incline your ear to my sayings. Let them not escape from your sight; keep them within your heart. For they are life to those who find them, and healing to all their flesh" (Proverbs 4:20–22). In Jesus' name, Amen.

Mastitis (Breastfeeding Difficulties) Healing Prayer

Father, You have created my body to feed my baby, and for that, I praise You. But an illness/infection is trying to rob me of this miracle, and I resist it right now in Jesus' name. Please heal me of the mastitis and all its symptoms, including the fever, chills, aches, fatigue and other flu-like symptoms resulting from this infection. Also, please bring relief to my breast from all inflammation, plugged ducts, engorgement, tenderness, cracked or bleeding nipples and pain. Holy Spirit, come. Help me rest, rest, rest and nurse, nurse, nurse to relieve the engorgement. "Can a woman forget her nursing child, that she should have no compassion on the son of her womb? Even these may forget, yet I will not forget you. Behold, I have engraved you on the palms of my hands" (Isaiah 49:15–16). In Jesus' name I pray, Amen.

Note: Also drink plenty of fluids and use massage and warm compresses for short periods of time to stimulate breast milk production, varying your baby's head position to empty each milk duct fully.

Menopause (and Perimenopause) Symptom Relief Prayer

Okay, Lord, I've had it. You did not create me to be tired, grumpy, unfocused, bloated or hot. Menopause is not a disease, but a transition. I call for grace to manifest right now to make this transition less uncomfortable and more enjoyable. I ask You to bring hormonal balance to my body, which will help ease the hot flashes, bloating, mood swings, water retention, insomnia, painful intercourse and skin changes. If You want me on bioidentical hormone replacement therapy (BHRT) that will reverse all of that, plus protect my heart and bone health, guide me to the right practitioner since I know that synthetic hormones are not healthy for me. Holy Spirit, come. I declare that I am not an old woman, but a vibrant woman of wisdom whose voice is needed in this next generation, so, Lord, energize me so that I might speak for You. "Then Jesus answered her, 'O woman, great is your faith! Be it done for you as you desire'" (Matthew 15:28). In Jesus' name, Amen.

Miscarriage Healing Prayer

O Father, the loss is almost too great to bear. We know by faith that we have not lost this child, because he or she is now with You. God, would You please care for him or her and send Your comfort to us here? We give you our hurt, pain and disappointment, but we also trust that You want to bless us with another baby. We will not give up [see the infertility prayer in this chapter]. Heal our bodies and hearts, and give us the emotional strength to begin again. Holy Spirit, come. We trust You for Your timing and know that when we hold our new baby, all this pain will seem but a breath. "He heals the brokenhearted and binds up their wounds" (Psalm 147:3). We ask it all in the name of Jesus, Amen.

Painful Menstrual Periods Healing Prayer

Lord, I am desperate for Your relief. Please help me and deliver me from this monthly misery. I believe You have a plan for me that does not involve debilitating pain, and I am determined to find peace for my body and entire reproductive system. In the mighty, healing name of Jesus Christ I rebuke and resist this crippling back pain and these cramps, upper leg pain, nausea, vomiting, light-headedness and immobility. I declare that if I have uterine fibroids, polycystic ovarian syndrome (PCOS), endometriosis [see the healing prayers for all those] or any other reproductive disorder, You are my Healer; therefore, there is health in my near future. Help me stick to the advice on this chapter's A-list and not make it difficult for You to answer this prayer! I declare that this is not "the curse," but that it is a blessing to be a woman, so I thank You. "For this light momentary affliction is preparing for us an eternal weight of glory beyond all comparison" (2 Corinthians 4:17). Holy Spirit, come. Thank You, Jesus. In Your name I pray it all, Amen.

Note: My middle daughter used to suffer from debilitating menstrual cycles in which she would faint, vomit, miss work and experience days of pain and misery. She was taking so much ibuprofen each month that it damaged the lining of her stomach and she wound up with leaky gut syndrome (see that prayer in chapter 17) and severe rectal bleeding, losing more than 30 pounds. She was down to 82 pounds, could no longer walk and was under my constant care, barely dodging hospitalization twice. By visiting the following link, you can see my published case study in which we resolved her situation in both her digestive and reproductive systems, resulting in total recovery and pain-free periods ever since: lauraharrissmith.com/testimonies. Relief is possible, and healing is yours!

Polycystic Ovarian Syndrome (PCOS) Healing Prayer

Jesus, I need a healing in my reproductive system, particularly my ovaries. Please touch both my ovaries and remove any enlargement, along with the small cysts that are trying to form on the outside edges. Father, this disorder is trying to leave me infertile, in pain and depressed, and I declare that I will be none of those! I will have children. I will be pain free. I will be full of joy! And I thank You for removing every other symptom, such as the heavy and irregular cycles, hair loss, absence of menstruation or ovulation, unwanted hair growth and acne. I also declare that I will not always battle my weight or become obese, but will find the healthy weight You desire for me. Holy Spirit, come. I receive Your grace right now to stick to the A-list advice in this chapter so that my reproductive system might thrive. I expect great things as a result of this obedience. Your Word says of You, "He gives the barren woman a home, making her the joyous mother of children. Praise the LORD!" (Psalm 113:9), and I claim that for myself. In the name of Jesus I pray, Amen.

Postpartum Depression Healing Prayer

Lord, You blessed us with this beautiful baby, but now my body and mind are overwhelmed. Please free me from the guilt over that, as well as the anxiety, mood swings, crying, panic attacks, anger, depression, irritability and fear. Give me freedom from the hopelessness, restlessness, insomnia, fatigue and unwanted thoughts. I also pray that You would help me manage my appetite so that my weight becomes balanced and healthy. I love this baby, Lord, and all my children, present and future. Holy Spirit, come. Restore to me the joy that I know is mine, and make me the happy mother (or father) of children. "For our heart is glad in him, because we trust in his holy name" (Psalm 33:21). In Jesus' name, Amen.

Premenstrual Syndrome (PMS) Healing Prayer

God, I can tell that my body is under the sway of hormonal changes, and I do not like the extreme changes that I see in myself and in my moods during this time of the month, every month. Holy Spirit, come. Would You please balance my hormones so that I can be more like myself and less like an impatient, easily offended version of myself that I don't recognize? Also, please bring me relief from the fatigue, swelling, bloating, appetite changes, breast tenderness, acne, weight gain, insomnia and the inability to concentrate. I also ask You to remove the pain and discomfort in my pelvis, back, joints, muscles and head. Remind me to steer clear of soy foods that mimic estrogen and only increase the hormonal imbalances, and help me to stick to this chapter's A-list for maximum reproductive health. I choose by faith not to dread these phases of my monthly cycles and to choose joy and positivity each time. "And without faith it is impossible to please him, for whoever would draw near to God must believe that he exists and that he rewards those who seek him" (Hebrews 11:6). In Jesus' name I pray, Amen.

Sexually Transmitted Diseases (STD) Healing Prayer

Jesus, I am turning to You, overwhelmed with this diagnosis and all the symptoms of this STD. If this is the result of my own sin, then, Lord, I ask You for forgiveness and healing in spirit, mind and body. If this is the result of my partner's sin that is now affecting and infecting me, then, Lord, I choose to forgive him or her, but I also ask for Your wisdom on how I should proceed with this relationship. Lord, whether it be chlamydia, gonorrhea, syphilis, genital herpes, human papillomavirus, HIV/AIDS or another STD, I know that You are bigger than these scary names and that You can make my body as good as new and restore my purity to me. Holy Spirit, come. I want to start over. I want to be clean. I know that only You can accomplish this. "Then they cried to the LORD in their trouble, and he delivered them from their distress. He sent out his word and healed them, and delivered them from their destruction" (Psalm 107:19–20). Thank You, Lord. It is in Your name that I pray it all, Amen.

Uterine Fibroids (Uterine Myoma) Healing Prayer

God, my reproductive system is in need of a touch from You, and I need You to bring healing to its most inward parts. Please cause any and all fibroids in my uterus to dissolve on their own so they would not cause my body any more distress, whether they be intramural, submucosal or subserosal fibroids. Holy Spirit, come. Take far away from me the pelvic pain, spotting and the abnormally heavy menstrual bleeding and prolonged periods. Lord, take away the abdominal distension, urination discomfort, leg pain and lower back cramping, and replace these with peace and comfort. No longer let fibroids stand in my way of becoming or staying pregnant, and I thank You in advance for the perfect hormonal balance to prevent any further fibroids from forming. "Come to me, all who labor and are heavy laden, and I will give you rest. Take my yoke upon you, and learn from me, for I am gentle and lowly in heart, and you will find rest for your souls. For my yoke is easy, and my burden is light" (Matthew 11:28–30). In Jesus' name I pray, Amen.

21

Skeletal System

Bones, Bone Marrow, Joints, Teeth, Ligaments, Cartilage

Declaration

I am ready to receive any needed healing for my skeletal system and then do whatever it takes to walk in divine health. I know that God does not make me sick, and I ask Him right now to show me the root of my condition, whether it be physical, emotional or spiritual. I am ready to pray the prayer of faith, reverse the curse and unleash the blessing. By God's grace, I will watch my words, maintain my miracle or wait on God's perfect timing for healing. Amen!

Skeletal System Blessing

I speak strength and wellness over that part of you that makes you look like you and gives you your unique **Skeletal System** facial geometry and other bodily characteristics—your skeletal system. I call for any broken, missing or misaligned bones to mend or regrow altogether in the name of Jesus. This includes the restoration and invigoration of all 206 bones that comprise the skeletal system, as well as the cartilage, tendons and ligaments that connect them. I speak strength to your spinal cord and its discs, for pain-free bending, sitting, standing, reclining and any other movement you desire, including the ability to worship freely and with liberty. I release full harmony between your skeletal system and your nervous system's nerves, and between your skeletal system and your cardiovascular system's blood vessels. Finally, I believe God for that bone health to extend to your teeth, which is an ultimate blessing to your digestive system. Let it be done according to your faith and in the mighty name of Jesus!

Visit lauraharrissmith.com/blessings for the video blessing.

Your Skeletal System's A-list

Avoid sugar, caffeine, white potatoes, soda, alcohol, excess salt, beef

Add nondairy calcium in the form of broccoli, kale, okra; beans, sweet potato; *exercise*

Allow calcium, magnesium taurate; vitamins C, D3, K2; trace minerals

Apply cedarwood, frankincense, wild orange, clove, basil, lavender oils

Anoint with oil daily and pray needed healing prayers and body system blessings

Ask your doctor or health care provider before making regimen changes

Your Skeletal System's Favorite . . .

Breakfast: fresh green juice, salsa eggs (scrambled eggs with tomato, onion, cilantro, cayenne powder)

Lunch: quinoa with bone broth, broccoli, carrots, cashews, turmeric; avocado with salmon or tuna

Dinner: cashew chicken with bone broth, garlic, grated ginger; cauliflower rice; green salad

Snack: celery and homemade salsa, hummus with cucumber slices or carrots; walnuts, flax, Brazil nuts, pumpkin seeds, strawberries, baked kale chips

Testimony

"I had surgery to repair a torn rotator cuff, torn bicep tendon and torn bicep. My PCP told me my poor shoulder resembled a pro-football injury. My surgeon advised that recovery would take six to eight weeks, and I spent the first five of that in typical postsurgery mode, just using my other arm and waiting to be pain free. Then I was sent Laura's body system blessings, and I began speaking them over myself at week five, particularly the skeletal system blessing. Exactly one week later, I had a follow-up visit with the orthopedic surgeon. He was blown away with my range of motion and lack of pain. Just to be cautious, he prescribed six weeks of physical therapy. I met with the therapist the following day. She went about her normal evaluation and told me that I would not need to return. She looked at me and said, 'You have rehabbed yourself. I am going to give you some exercises to do at home and let your doctor know.' In addition to my recovery that the therapist described as 'astounding,' since reading all these body system blessings over myself daily, I have had an intense overall sense of well-being. Everything in my body seems to be firing on all cylinders, as it all was created to do. That may not seem to be such a huge deal in and of itself, but at 64 years of age, I am loving it." ~Elaine

After reading the blessings and prayers, send all testimonies large and small to healing@lauraharrissmith.com.

Skeletal System Healing Prayers

Abscessed Tooth Healing Prayer

Lord, I am in great need of Your relief. Please calm and heal the infection so that the source of the pain might be removed entirely. I receive Your touch right now to alleviate the pain in the root, jaw and tooth, and I ask You to heal even the cavity itself. Holy Spirit, come. As the infection goes, I know that the fever and chills will go, along with the pus, bad breath and swollen lymph nodes. "Then the LORD put out his hand and touched my mouth" (Jeremiah 1:9). I ask it all in the healing name of Jesus, Amen.

Broken Bone (Fracture) Healing Prayer

Note: I have had the Lord heal a broken rib for me in minutes, as proven by "before and after" X-rays. Please see the pneumothorax prayer in the respiratory system chapter for the full testimony.

Father, I know You are able to heal a bone as quickly as it broke. I believe in Your healing Word, Lord, and I ask You to help my body line up with it right now. Holy Spirit, come. I declare that bones will mend supernaturally and that my pain will begin to cease even as I pray this. Also take care of any bruising, swelling, tenderness, bleeding or other issues with my muscular system that resulted from this injury. Thank You that it was not any worse! "And Peter said to him, 'Aeneas, Jesus Christ heals you; rise and make your bed.' And immediately he rose" (Acts 9:34). I pray it in Your name, Jesus. Amen.

Bursitis Healing Prayer

Father, I should not feel this old. I should not feel so stiff. I am asking You to touch the fluid-filled pads that are cushioning my joints (the bursae) and bring healing. Whether they are in my arm, hip, knee, shoulder, elbow or elsewhere, heal me of the inflammation, swelling, tenderness and pain that is interfering with their ability to function as they should. Help me be pain free whether resting or moving, and especially during repetitive movements. If there was an underlying injury, please repair what was damaged there, too. Holy Spirit, come. I know You do not want me to hurt every day. "The thief comes only to steal and kill and destroy. I came that they may have life and have it abundantly" (John 10:10). In Jesus' name, Amen.

Gout Healing Prayer

Jesus, I hurt. I am asking You to touch my joints and set my entire skeletal system free from this pain and inflammation. Please rid me of the redness, stiffness and the physical deformities. Remove the swelling in my joints, particularly my big toe, and bring me relief in my ankles, feet and knees. Please prevent any further uric acid from crystalizing and depositing itself in my joints, and deliver me from every trace of arthritis, God. May my nights be peaceful and my sleep be sweet. Holy Spirit, come. "And behold a hand touched me, and lifted me up upon my knees, and upon the joints of my hands" (Daniel 10:10 DRA). I pray these things in Your name, Amen.

Herniated Disc Healing Prayer

God, I know that You can touch my spinal column right now and alleviate the pain. I have a few options of different remedies I can try for relief, but none compare to a touch from You, and I do want You alone to get all the glory. Please heal the spinal disc(s) bulging and pushing through the crack in my spine's exterior casing. Please remove the pain in my arms, back, legs and feet, and the muscle weakness in general. Also bring relief to the muscle spasms and overactive reflexes, Lord. Holy Spirit, come. Please heal me from this numbness, tingling, burning, stiffness and the pins-and-needles sensations. "Thus says the Lord GOD to these bones: Behold, I will cause breath to enter you, and you shall live" (Ezekiel 37:5). Thank You, Lord, because I do want to live . . . and live pain free. In Your name I pray, Amen.

Osteoarthritis Healing Prayer

"Have compassion on me, LORD, for I am weak. Heal me, LORD, for my bones are in agony" (Psalm 6:2 NLT). Lord, this prayer almost says it all. Please remove all inflammation from every finger, wrist, hand, toe, ankle, arm, leg, hip, knee and every joint in my body, God. Please give me back my range of motion and flexibility, as well as muscle strength that allows me to walk again with ease. Energize me to get rid of the fatigue and stiffness, and please reduce any bony outgrowth that has taken place in my fingers and toes. I will walk! I will rise! I will write and type and do anything else I need to do to live an active life. Holy Spirit, come. And remind me to adhere to this chapter's A-list advice so that my skeletal system might not experience these flares ever again. I pray it in the name of Jesus, Amen.

Osteogenesis Imperfecta (Brittle Bone Disease) Healing Prayer

Jesus, only You can cause my body to begin producing more collagen so that my bones are better nourished. Literally rewrite my DNA so that my genes are overridden and I begin to grow stronger instead of weaker. Heal me of any current bone fractures, the bone tissue formation, bruising, calluses and stiffness. Let the healing continue to my frame itself, whether it be bowed legs, an enlarged head, physical deformities or even scoliosis [see the scoliosis healing prayer in this chapter]. I thank You that any hearing loss is going to be reversed and that my eyes will be bright again and reflect the healing You have done for me. Holy Spirit, come. Whether I have broken just a few bones, or literally hundreds, as happens to some with this illness, please protect me from any future breaks. "For the Lord protects the bones of the righteous; not one of them is broken!" (Psalm 34:20 NLT). In Jesus' name I pray, Amen.

Osteoporosis Healing Prayer

Lord, my bones need rejuvenation. Please cause my body to renew and replace with new and healthy bone tissue the old bone tissue that is constantly being absorbed. Defy what is possible in the natural, O God! Please give me back my height, my posture and my ability to live an active life without fear. Please mend any fractures I have had so that there is never a rebreak in that same spot, or in any other. Holy Spirit, come. And help me desire the foods on this chapter's A-list so that my bones might prosper as I age. "And the LORD will guide you continually and satisfy your desire in scorched places and make your bones strong; and you shall be like a watered garden, like a spring of water, whose waters do not fail" (Isaiah 58:11). In Jesus' name I pray these things, Amen.

Rheumatoid Arthritis (RA) Healing Prayer

Jesus, I realize that RA is different than osteoarthritis since it is more of an autoimmune disorder and less about general wear and tear on my joints, but all I know is that I hurt. Holy Spirit, come. Would You please touch my body and reverse the curse of arthritis? Please cause my immune system to stop attacking my own tissue, including my joints. Please heal me from the joint pain, fatigue, swelling, numbness, muscle pain, back discomfort and even any anemia. Heal my skin, Jesus, from all lumps and redness. "A joyful heart is good medicine, but a crushed spirit dries up the bones" (Proverbs 17:22). Thank You for Your healing, O God! In Jesus' name I pray, Amen.

Scoliosis Healing Prayer

Lord, only You can supernaturally touch my spine and cause it to straighten. I am ready to have even shoulders, a level waist and symmetrical hips. I declare that my spine will not twist or rotate, and that the curvature will begin to straighten and improve, starting now. Jesus, if there is an underlying condition such as a neuromuscular condition, an injury or a birth defect, I truly believe those are not too difficult for You to heal. And if this is an inherited family trait, please both heal me and prevent my children from having this curvature—or heal them, too, if they already have it. Holy Spirit, come. Help me nourish my entire skeletal system with the foods on this chapter's A-list. "This will be healing for your body and strengthening for your bones" (Proverbs 3:8 HCSB). In the name of Jesus, Amen.

TMJ (Temporomandibular Joint Syndrome) Healing Prayer

Heavenly Father, my jaw, mouth and teeth ache. I don't believe that You want me to struggle with TMJ forever, so I am asking You to heal me. Holy Spirit, come. Touch the temporomandibular joints in my jaw, please, and give me relief and restoration for the opening and closing of my mouth, and for chewing, singing and even laughing. Keep my jaw from ever locking and from the discomfort of the clicking, clenching and grating sensations. Please heal any bone erosion that has occurred and realign anything that is out of place, Lord. Heal any arthritis that has set in or any cartilage that has been damaged by it. "The light of the eyes rejoices the heart, and good news refreshes the bones" (Proverbs 15:30). In the name of Jesus, I thank You and pray, Amen.

22

Muscular System
Muscles

Declaration

I am ready to receive any needed healing for my muscular system and then do whatever it takes to walk in divine health. I know that God does not make me sick, and I ask Him right now to show me the root of my condition, whether it be physical, emotional or spiritual. I am ready to pray the prayer of faith, reverse the curse and unleash the blessing. By God's grace, I will watch my words, maintain my miracle or wait on God's perfect timing for healing. Amen!

Muscular System Blessing

On top of the blessing spoken over your skeletal system, I now release the benefit of perfect health and strength to the more than seven hundred named muscles that comprise your muscular system. Without them, **Muscular System** movement is impossible, but with them and their proper nerve connection, they can and will take you wherever you need to go. I speak complete and total mobility over you. All of your skeletal muscular tissue, blood vessels, tendons and nerves are in their proper places and are working together to make you move pain free. Whether it be an involuntary muscle such as your visceral or cardiac muscles, or a voluntary muscle such as all your skeletal muscles, I speak perfect health over them all. Get moving! Let it be done according to your faith and in the mighty name of Jesus!

Visit lauraharrissmith.com/blessings for the video blessing.

Your Muscular System's A-List

Avoid wheat, sodas, sugar, alcohol, pork, chips, cereals; *dehydration*

Add eggs, beans; grass-fed beef, organic chicken, salmon (if meat eater)

Allow vitamins B complex, C, D3; calcium, selenium, iron, fish oil, magnesium taurate

Apply frankincense, lavender, clove, eucalyptus, cypress, sandalwood oils

Anoint with oil daily and pray needed healing prayers and body system blessings

Ask your doctor or health care provider before making regimen changes

Your Muscular System's Favorite . . .

Breakfast: almond butter with banana; omelet with egg, spinach, red bell pepper, broccoli, turmeric

Lunch: egg drop soup with bone broth, eggs, chives, gluten-free soy sauce, turmeric, salt, white pepper

Dinner: navy beans in bone broth with tomatoes, spinach, potatoes, onion, pink salt; beet chips

Snack: apples, oranges, berries, bananas, walnuts, cashews, roasted chickpeas (toss 1 drained can with olive oil, chili powder, pink salt and roast at 350° for 30 minutes)

Testimony

"God began to show me which areas of my body needed to receive the blessings, and I started speaking the blessings and declarations over them since I had had severe neck pain for more than a month. The day after, the pain in my neck was instantly healed." ~Supiati

After reading the blessings and prayers, send all testimonies large and small to healing@lauraharrissmith.com.

Muscular System Healing Prayers

Carpal Tunnel Syndrome Healing Prayer

Jesus, I am stretching my hands up to You right now for healing. Please bring relief to the pinched nerve(s) causing this numbness and tingling in my wrist(s). I need these hands to complete my work, and I know You do not want me to live a life of clumsiness, hand weakness, wrist discomfort or arm pain. Holy Spirit, come. Thank You in advance for healing me so that I might do my work by day and so that I might rest better at night. "Then he said to the man, 'Stretch out your hand.' And the man stretched it out, and it was restored, healthy like the other" (Matthew 12:13). In Jesus' name I pray all of this, Amen.

Fibromyalgia Healing Prayer

Father, I am convinced that You do not want me to live a life of pain, whether in my back, abdomen, legs, neck or any other portion of my muscular system. Holy Spirit, come. Please take from me the chronic mood swings, fatigue, forgetfulness, sleeplessness and lack of concentration. Ease my GI tract so that I am no longer nauseous, gassy or constipated. Lord, please bring me relief from being sore all over, and from the often sharp and severe pain. I don't want to be anxious. I don't want to be nervous. I don't want to be depressed or battle headaches, joint stiffness or sensitivity to cold anymore. I know You have a life for me that is free of fibromyalgia, and I will nourish my body with foods from this chapter's A-list so I do not hinder You answering my prayers. "And he called to him his twelve disciples and gave them authority over unclean spirits, to cast them out, and to heal every disease and every affliction" (Matthew 10:1). I pray it all in Your name, Amen.

Lower Back Pain (Lumbago) Healing Prayer

Lord, these strains and sprains are agonizing, but I know You are able to heal them! I believe You want me to be able to rise, walk, bend, lift, stand up straight and even exercise. Please touch the muscles near the base of my spine and mend whatever needs mending. Also remove from me the numbness, muscle spasms, pins and needles, and any joint dysfunction. I also trust You to correct any deferred pain in my hips, legs, waist and pelvis. Holy Spirit, come. Thank You in advance for Your healing touch. "For we walk by faith, not by sight" (2 Corinthians 5:7). In Jesus' name I pray, Amen.

Multiple Sclerosis (MS) Healing Prayer

O Great Physician, I know this disorder involves my immune system attacking my nervous system, but all I know is that I feel it daily in my muscular system. So I am turning to You for deliverance from this painful cycle. Please cause my immune system to stop attacking the protective myelin sheaths in my nervous system that control all my muscles and their nerves. Command that myelin to regrow, and command those very nerves to heal from any damage they have incurred. Please bring me relief from the weakness, numbness, tingling, tremor and even the electric-shock sensations that sometimes accompany my neck movements. Heal my eyes, O God, and remove the double vision, vision loss and overall eye pain and strain. Holy Spirit, come. I declare that I will be able to walk steadily, speak clearly, control my bladder, bowel and sexual function, and that I will move without dizziness or weariness. "But they who wait for the LORD shall renew their strength; they shall mount up with wings like eagles; they shall run and not be weary; they shall walk and not faint" (Isaiah 40:31). In Jesus' name, Amen.

Muscle Spasms / Cramps Healing Prayer

Lord, I am ready to be pain free and to have my muscles stop involuntarily contracting night and day. Please touch my muscular and nervous systems and cause them to work together better to alleviate this discomfort, whether it be in my legs, back, neck, shoulders, arms, hips or fingers. Please remove the swelling, redness, weakness, pain and skin changes that sometimes result. Holy Spirit, come. May I be mindful of abiding by the foods on this chapter's A-list so that I might nourish my muscles and not harm or deprive them. "Look carefully then how you walk, not as unwise but as wise" (Ephesians 5:15). In Jesus' name I pray this, Amen.

Muscular Dystrophy (MD) Healing Prayer

Jesus, a diagnosis of MD is daunting, but in the end muscular dystrophy is just a name, and You have the name above all names. So I am turning to You for healing, Lord. First, heal the abnormal genes and mutations that are leading to my muscle degeneration, and begin the restoration process on any muscles that have already atrophied. Balm of Gilead, I receive You into the very core of my muscles so that they might be strengthened, not hang loosely, and never shorten. Holy Spirit, come. Please deliver me of any other MD symptoms such as cardiomyopathy, constipation, difficulty swallowing, scoliosis and shallow breathing. In short, please cause my muscular, nervous, digestive, skeletal and cardiovascular systems to work together to provide healing for my entire body. "But Peter said, 'I have no silver and gold, but what I do have I give to you. In the name of Jesus Christ of Nazareth, rise up and walk!'" (Acts 3:6). I pray it all in Your name, Amen.

Polio Healing Prayer

Heavenly Father, please strengthen my body so that it is resistant to the poliovirus and defeats it within my body. Please touch my entire muscular and nervous systems and bring healing wherever needed. I declare that I will not live a life of weakness, faintness, fever, nausea and physical paralysis. I pray protection over myself and my loved ones from any transmittal of the poliovirus in food and water, or through direct contact with an infected person. I do not believe You want me to spend my life on bedrest with portable ventilators and pain relievers, so I turn to You for help. Holy Spirit, come. I proclaim that I will be entirely restored and that my muscles will grow as needed and become strong. "Walk as children of light" (Ephesians 5:8). I will! In Your name I pray this, Amen.

Restless Legs Syndrome (RLS) Healing Prayer

Lord, I am ready to rest without having my legs race! Please heal me of this nearly irresistible urge to move my legs when I am reclining. Bring peace to every charley horse and to all tingling, burning and restless jerking. RLS has interfered with my sleep for too long, and as a result it has caused me to be sleep deprived and fatigued during the day. Holy Spirit, come. Heal this and help me follow the A-list advice given in this chapter. Also remind me to hydrate myself by consuming plenty of water each day and by taking a good magnesium taurate supplement, which has been proven to help calm those nerves. "Your word is a lamp to my feet and a light to my path" (Psalm 119:105). In Jesus' name I pray, Amen.

Tendinitis Healing Prayer

Jesus, the tissue connecting some of my muscles to my bones has become inflamed, and I am coming to You to heal it. You can touch where no other finger can go, and I know You don't want me to live such a life of discomfort. Whether it's tennis elbow, golfer's elbow, Achilles tendinitis, swimmer's shoulder, patellar tendinitis, de Quervain's tenosynovitis or some other form, I am laying my hand on the location right now and asking You to heal it. "They will lay their hands on the sick, and they will recover" (Mark 16:18). Holy Spirit, come. I believe You are beginning my healing even now. In Jesus' name I pray all of this, Amen.

Whiplash Healing Prayer

Father, this whiplash injury has caused me some unexpected pain, particularly in my neck, shoulders, back and arms. Holy Spirit, come. Please heal me of the dizziness, vertigo, difficulty focusing and tenderness. I also ask that You watch over me as I sleep and give me true rest that is free of muscle spasms, headaches, pins-and-needles sensations and pain. I also declare that I will not develop any sleep disorders through this and that my sleep will not be disturbed, delayed or decreased. "Many are the afflictions of the righteous, but the LORD delivers him out of them all" (Psalm 34:19). In Your name I pray, Amen.

23

Immune System

Bone Marrow, Thymus, Glands

Note: The twenty diseases listed in this chapter and the next can manifest in any body system, but since strong immune and lymphatic systems are required for healing all twenty of them, I placed them under these systems. For instance, staph can manifest anywhere in the body, but it is listed under the immune system as a general means of categorization. And cancer can manifest anywhere in the body, but it is listed under the lymphatic system for the same reason. It will take healing in both these body systems—the immune and the lymphatic—to overcome these twenty diseases.

Declaration

I am ready to receive any needed healing for my immune system and then do whatever it takes to walk in

Immune System

divine health. I know that God does not make me sick, and I ask Him right now to show me the root of my condition, whether it be physical, emotional or spiritual. I am ready to pray the prayer of faith, reverse the curse and unleash the blessing. By God's grace, I will watch my words, maintain my miracle or wait on God's perfect timing for healing. Amen!

Immune System Blessing

I release a warrior blessing over your immune system so that it would be able to detect and defeat any and all germs, viruses, bacteria and even chronic illnesses that would try to invade your healthy body and bring disease. I bless and release wellness over the intricate relationship between your bone marrow, thymus, tonsils, lymph nodes, skin and your digestive system, which houses more than 70 percent of your immune system. Your immunities are strong! You will foster this with proper rest, nutrition, exercise and abstention from the things that the Holy Spirit shows you to omit concerning your body, mind or spirit. Between your strong immune system and the Holy Spirit's protection, you are doubly protected from all diseases and disorders. Let it be done according to your faith and in the mighty name of Jesus!

Visit lauraharrissmith.com/blessings for the video blessing.

Your Immune System's A-list

Avoid sugar, sodas, red meat, fried foods, dairy, processed foods; *stress*

Add citrus, garlic, ginger, turmeric, green tea; *daily exercise, 8 hours sleep*

Allow a strong probiotic; zinc, selenium; vitamins B6, C, C3, E; folic acid

Apply oregano, tea tree, lemon, lemongrass, lavender, cinnamon, clove oils

Anoint with oil daily and pray needed healing prayers and body system blessings

Ask your doctor or health care provider before making regimen changes

Your Immune System's Favorite . . .

Breakfast: "red" eggs (eggs scrambled with diced tomato, red pepper, red onion, cayenne)

Lunch: Skinny Pasta or The Only Bean gluten-free edamame pasta with tomato sauce, veggies

Dinner: lemon-ginger cashew stir-fry with chicken or tofu, broccoli, cilantro, cashews, ginger, lemon

Snack: fresh carrot and beet juice, citrus fruits, sunflower seeds, red peppers, tomatoes, red onion, kiwi, papaya, broccoli, spinach, garlic, turmeric, ginger, almonds, green tea

Testimony

"Every year during this season, I'm in bed sick with some kind of sinus infection or viral infection. I haven't been sick at all this season after reading Laura's immune system blessing! Most of my doctors have told me that I have a weak immune system because of all the antibiotics and steroids I have been on since I was a baby. I have tried for years to do more natural stuff to build up my immune system, but when we go on vacations I usually get sick as well. Recently, however, I didn't get sick at all on our trip! I had medicine from my doctor along as a precaution, but I didn't need it! I was so grateful and was praising God!" ~Velvet

After reading the blessings and prayers, send all testimonies large and small to healing@lauraharrissmith.com.

Immune System Healing Prayers

Allergies (Food, Environmental, Chemical, Animal and Seasonal) Healing Prayer

Jesus, my immune system is confused and has identified a particular substance as harmful to me, when it actually is not. Please bring order and discernment to my immune system and cause it to pick its battles better, resulting in fewer allergies. I thank You in advance for healing me of the varying symptoms like congestion; sneezing; red, watery eyes and itchy nose, eyes and roof of mouth. Please reduce any and all swelling, whether it be in my eyes, throat, face, lips, tongue, limbs or trunk, and please eliminate all hives from my outsides and insides and calm my skin's itchy rashes. Heal all coughs and wheezing, and protect me from anaphylactic shock. I also receive Your invitation to make the changes necessary for better health, adhering to this chapter's A-list nutritional advice. Holy Spirit, come. "Jesus saw the huge crowd as He stepped from the boat, and He had compassion on them and healed their sick" (Matthew 14:14 NLT). In Jesus' name, Amen.

Candida (Thrush / Yeast Infection) Healing Prayer

Lord, I need You to help me eradicate this fungal infection that has invaded my body. Please remove from me the digestive problems, hormone imbalance, sweet cravings and joint pain. I also ask You to revive me from this exhaustion and brain fog, and to fortify my weak immune system that is resulting in all the sinus and allergy issues and UTIs. Remove all traces of this infection in my mouth, genitals, digestive tract, skin, nails and bloodstream. Holy Spirit, come. Help me implement immediately those foods on this chapter's A-list, while also abstaining from all wheat and sugar, which this fungal infection feeds on. I am following You, trusting You and pressing in to healing. "For he had healed many, so that all who had diseases pressed around him to touch him" (Mark 3:10). In Your name, Lord, Amen.

Flu (Influenza) Healing Prayer

Holy Spirit, come. My body is aching, and I have places to go and people to see! Jesus, heal me from the virus that has invaded my body and produced these chills, fever, headache, fatigue and body aches [for stomach flu, see the nausea/vomiting prayer in chapter 17]. Please remove the head congestion, runny nose, cough, chest pressure, sore throat, sneezing and shortness of breath. As my immune system fights this infection off with Your help, grace my lymphatic system to drain it off quickly and without incident. "For I am the LORD, your healer" (Exodus 15:26). In Jesus' name, Amen.

HIV/AIDS Healing Prayer

O Great God, this diagnosis is intimidating, and I can feel it in my heart and see it on the faces of those who love me. But I also know You love me, so, Lord, the only face I want to see right now is Yours. You are my Healer. You are my first love. "Come, let us return to the LORD; for he has torn us, that he may heal us; he has struck us down, and he will bind us up" (Hosea 6:1). Lord, remove this infection from my body, I pray, and take with it the initial flu-like symptoms, fever, sore throat, cough and fatigue. Take away the nausea, abdominal discomfort, diarrhea and vomiting, and replace them with a healthy appetite and weight gain. Please heal me of the various pains—when I swallow, when I'm swollen and when I'm sweating—and grace my lymphatic system to drain what my improving immune system is fighting off for me. Touch my skin and make it new again. Free it from all blemishes and red blotches, and heal my mouth from all ulcers and thrush, Jesus. Holy Spirit, come. You have my full attention and my full heart. It's in the healing name of Jesus I pray this, Amen.

Lupus Healing Prayer

Heavenly Father, my immune system is confused and is attacking its own tissues, so I need You to speak truth to it and cause it to cease. I will not live my life in chronic pain. Not in my joints, not in my muscles, not in my chest and not when breathing. Please remove from me this anxiety, depression, headache, anemia and fatigue, while also healing me from the light sensitivity, swelling, water retention, hair loss, mouth ulcers and rash. Holy Spirit, come. I am too young to feel this old, so I call for an end to all inflammation today, in the name of Jesus. I also accept Your invitation to make the changes necessary for better health and to adhere to this chapter's A-list nutritional advice. "But for this purpose I have raised you up, to show you my power, so that my name may be proclaimed in all the earth" (Exodus 9:16). Be glorified through me, Lord. In Your name, Amen.

Mononucleosis (Epstein-Barr Virus) Healing Prayer

Father, what started with body aches and headaches has become much more serious, and I need Your healing. Please heal me of this fever, muscle pain, fatigue, sore throat and swollen tonsils, weakness, abdominal pain and skin rash. Please protect my liver and spleen from swelling. Also touch my lymph nodes all over my body so that their swelling might reduce as they usher this Epstein-Barr virus out of my body through my lymphatic system. Holy Spirit, come. Please bolster my immune system so that it might resist related illnesses such as type 1 diabetes, rheumatoid arthritis (RA), inflammatory bowel disease (IBD), systemic lupus erythematosus (SLE), multiple sclerosis (MS), juvenile idiopathic arthritis (JIA), and celiac disease. "And when Jesus entered Peter's house, he saw his mother-in-law lying sick with a fever. He touched her hand, and the fever left her, and she rose and began to serve him" (Matthew 8:14–15). In Jesus' name, let it be the same for me. Amen.

MRSA Superbug Healing Prayer

O Great Physician, only You can heal this strain of bacteria that has invaded my body. It is distinct from other staph infections in that it has become resistant to almost all antibiotics, so You are literally my only hope. Please bring relief to me from these painful boils and skin sores, especially the pus-filled pockets. Protect my joints, bones, heart valves, lungs and even my bloodstream from the harm this infection seeks to cause. Reinforce my immune system to fight, fight, fight further outbreaks, and fortify my spiritual immunities against those things that keep me from keeping my eyes on You and Your commandments. "It will become fine dust over the whole land of Egypt, and festering boils will break out on people and animals throughout the land" (Exodus 9:9 NIV), but "If you will carefully obey the LORD your God, do what he sees to be right, listen to his commandments, and keep all his statutes, then I won't inflict on you all the diseases that I inflicted on the Egyptians, because I am the LORD your healer" (Exodus 15:26 ISV). Holy Spirit, come. In the name of Jesus I pray, Amen.

Parasites (Parasitism) Healing Prayer

Jesus, another organism is trying to take up residency in my body, but I know that You can see it, remove it and bring healing. Please remove these painful symptoms of abdominal pain, diarrhea, vomiting and appetite changes. Please also heal me from the skin rashes and bumps, allergies and anemia. I also ask You to eliminate this fever, and the general weakness and discomfort. Lord, whether it is an endoparasite, epiparasite, ectoparasite, protozoa or helminth, please remove it and replace it with good health. Holy Spirit, come. Strengthen my immune system to finish what You begin. "For I consider that the sufferings of this present time are not worth comparing with the glory that is to be revealed to us" (Romans 8:18). In the name of Jesus, Amen.

Q Fever Healing Prayer

God, this very rare bacterium has found its way into my body through an infected animal, and I am asking You to heal me. Bolster my immune system to fight it off, and please relieve me of all symptoms including the fatigue, headache, nausea and shortness of breath. I also thank You that as You bring healing, this fever will decrease and my chills, sweats and achy muscles will subside. Holy Spirit, come. Thank You for hearing my prayer. "And Jesus went throughout all the cities and villages, teaching in their synagogues and proclaiming the gospel of the kingdom and healing every disease and every affliction" (Matthew 9:35). In Jesus' name, Amen.

Zoster (Shingles) Healing Prayer

Lord Jesus, the pain has been almost unbearable, but I know that as I turn to You, You will lead me to healing. Please deliver my body from the herpes zoster virus and heal me of its symptoms, such as the rash, blisters, ulcers, scabs and the burning and itching. As You remove these discomforts, I declare that they will never manifest in my body again. I also declare that after the rash is gone, I will not experience postherpetic neuralgia (the post-rash pain). Holy Spirit, come. I trust You for total healing. "Whatever you ask in my name, this I will do, that the Father may be glorified in the Son" (John 14:13). In Jesus' mighty name, Amen.

24

Lymphatic System

Spleen, Lymph Nodes, Ducts, Tonsils

Note: As I mentioned at the beginning of chapter 23, the twenty diseases listed in these two chapters can manifest in any body system, but since strong immune and lymphatic systems are required for healing all twenty of them, I placed them under these systems. It will take healing in both these body systems—the immune and the lymphatic—to overcome the twenty diseases mentioned in these two chapters.

Declaration

I am ready to receive any needed healing for my lymphatic system and then do whatever it takes to walk in divine health. I know that God does not make me sick, and I ask Him right now to show me the root of my condition, whether it be physical, emotional or spiritual. I am **Lymphatic System** ready to pray the prayer of faith, reverse the curse and unleash the blessing. By God's grace, I will watch my words, maintain my miracle or wait on God's perfect timing for healing. Amen!

Lymphatic System Blessing

As I speak this blessing over you and you begin to nourish your lymphatic system with the foods that make it thrive, your body's main cleansing mechanism—your lymphatic system—is about to receive its own natural and supernatural cleansing. This restored lymphatic system's spleen, nodes and ducts will drain well, keep your blood perfectly healthy, detox your body from impure toxins and keep your digestive tract on track. You are going to hear your body urging you to refrain from processed foods, sugary foods, bad oils and even dairy foods that slow lymph down. You will also quickly see changes in any sluggishness, stiffness, indigestion, mucus or frequent illnesses you struggle with. With God's supernatural touch and your dietary cooperation, along with hot showers, massage and exercise, your lymphatic system will be a lean, mean cleaning machine! Let it be done according to your faith and in the mighty name of Jesus.

Visit lauraharrissmith.com/blessings for the video blessing.

Your Lymphatic System's A-list

Avoid dairy, wheat, soy, shellfish, junk food, low-quality animal products

Add citrus, greens, cinnamon, black pepper; *body brushing, massage*

Allow fish oil, goldenseal, milk thistle, charcoal, daily morning lemon water

Apply lemon, grapefruit, orange, frankincense, peppermint, cypress oils

Anoint with oil daily and pray needed healing prayers and body system blessings

Ask your doctor or health care provider before making regimen changes

Your Lymphatic System's Favorite . . .

Breakfast: smoothie—2 cups watermelon, ½ lemon, ½ cup cilantro, 1 tablespoon aloe vera juice, ½ teaspoon stevia

Lunch: pinto beans and cauliflower rice mixed with tomato, avocado, garlic, olive oil; arugula salad

Dinner: sautéed chicken (or tofu) with sesame seeds, grated ginger, garlic, chicken stock, ½ teaspoon guar gum powder, gluten-free soy sauce

Snack: citrus, pumpkin seeds, sunflower seeds, walnuts, almonds, Brazil nuts, cashews, hazelnuts, cranberries, other berries

Testimony

"Laura's recommendations for foods I should avoid to allow better lymphatic system function—dairy, in particular—caused an "aha!" moment for me. I have been getting tension headaches for years that include painful knots in my neck. I've never been able to pinpoint what might be causing them. When I avoided dairy completely for a few days and then slipped up and had some cheesecake, it quickly became clear to me that the headaches are caused by the dairy clogging up my lymphatic system, particularly in my neck. I love the idea of praying over specific body systems for healing and guidance." ~Priscilla

After reading the blessings and prayers, send all testimonies large and small to healing@lauraharrissmith.com.

Lymphatic System Healing Prayers

Bites and Stings—Snake, Spider, Lice, Chigger, Insect, Wasp, Bee, Flea, Bedbug, Animal (of Any Kind), Scorpion, Tick (Non-Lyme)—Healing Prayer

Father, heal me of the pain and discomfort from this bite or sting. Remove from my system any poison, venom or harmful substances that have been injected into my bloodstream as a result. Cause the poison to disappear through the draining routes of a strong lymphatic system, in Jesus' name. Soothe the skin of any broken or swollen places, and calm the pain and any reactions like itching, burning, swelling, congestion, coughing, difficulty breathing and increased heart rate. Holy Spirit, come. Protect me from anaphylactic shock now and in the hours to come. "They will pick up serpents with their hands; and if they drink any deadly poison, it will not hurt them"(Mark 16:18). In the mighty name of Jesus I pray, Amen.

Cancer Healing Prayer

O Great God, it's cancer. Steady me in Your loving embrace, and remind me of Your great healing ability and Your great care for me. Cure me of this cellular disorder where some abnormal cells have divided and multiplied quickly, trying to destroy my healthy body tissue. Lord, wherever the cancer is—whether in the breast, blood, bone, prostate, colon, ovaries, stomach, bladder, brain, esophagus, pituitary, eyes, mouth, gallbladder, kidneys, liver, pancreas, stomach, uterus, thyroid, rectum, testicles, lungs, lymph or on the skin—it is just a name, and You have the name above all names. Holy Spirit, come. I declare that my immune and lymphatic systems will work together to bolster my healthy cells and cause them to grow and win. I also accept Your invitation to make the changes necessary for better health and to adhere to this chapter's A-list nutritional advice. "Indeed he was ill, near to death. But God had mercy on him, and not only on him but on me also, lest I should have sorrow upon sorrow" (Philippians 2:27). Thank You, Jesus. In Your name, Amen.

Leukemia Healing Prayer

Jesus, You are not afraid of leukemia, but leukemia is afraid of You. You alone can abolish it from my body by Your command, and I am asking You to do just that. Remove this cancer from my blood and take with it the weakness, dizziness, appetite changes and unhealthy weight loss. Please heal the nosebleeds, infections, shortness of breath, red spots on my skin, easy bruising, mouth ulcers and overall fatigue. Holy Spirit, come. I know that the fever means my immune system is fighting, and that the swollen lymph nodes mean my lymphatic system is trying to drain this sickness from my body. So for both of those discomforts, I thank You and declare that my body will win. My body will heal. My body will live. "He asked life of you; you gave it to him, length of days forever and ever" (Psalm 21:4). In the name of Jesus Christ, Amen.

Lyme Disease Healing Prayer

Great Physician, I need You to touch my body and remove this bacteria, Borrelia burgdorferi, from my bloodstream. This tiny tick bite is attempting to wreak havoc on my body, my mind, my finances and my future, but I declare in Your name that it will not win. Healing is mine. I rebuke these symptoms of fatigue, stiffness, joint pain, swelling and muscle pain. Holy Spirit, come. I declare that my immune system is fighting hard (as evidenced by the fever), and my lymphatic system will drain away the bacteria quickly. I also declare that this bull's-eye rash will go, as well as soreness around the site of the bite. I have faith in Your healing power, Lord. "'For I know the plans I have for you,' declares the LORD, 'plans to prosper you and not to harm you, plans to give you hope and a future'" (Jeremiah 29:11 NIV). In Your name, Lord, Amen.

Lymphedema Healing Prayer

L ord, in Your name I command this swelling in my limbs that is caused by a lymphatic system blockage to reduce. I also proclaim that my immune and circulatory systems are cooperating and working together toward that reduction, allowing the water retention, discomfort and pain to stop. Holy Spirit, come. Order my steps so that I will fit in time for exercise and massage, and grace me to stick to this chapter's A-list advice so that my lymphatic system will reach optimum health. "And He sent them out to proclaim the kingdom of God and to perform healing" (Luke 9:2 NASB). In the healing name of Jesus, Amen.

Malaria Healing Prayer

H eavenly Father, somehow, this very rare disease, which is caused by a mosquito bite, has intruded upon my body. My immune system is fighting hard, as evidenced by the fever and chills, and my lymphatic system is trying to help, as proven by the sweating and swollen lymph nodes. Holy Spirit, come. Remove from me the diarrhea, vomiting and nausea, as well as the abdominal pain and fatigue. Calm this fast heart rate, headache and confusion, and energize me with clarity and healing. I rebuke this infection in the name of Jesus and receive total healing in His name. "And they overcame him by the blood of the Lamb, and by the word of their testimony; and they loved not their lives unto the death" (Revelation 12:11 KJV). In Jesus' name, Amen.

Measles (Rubeola) Healing Prayer

G od, this very rare viral infection has found me [or my child], and I am asking You for healing. Please bring relief from the fever, fatigue and of course the red, blotchy skin rash. Ease the inflamed eyes and the general flu-like symptoms of muscle aches, sore throat, cough, runny nose and headache [see the pink eye healing prayer in chapter 12 and the flu prayer in chapter 23]. Please bring relief from the diarrhea and loss of appetite, and restore health, as only You can do. "'Again I say to you, if two of you agree on earth about anything they ask, it will be done for them by my Father in heaven'" (Matthew 18:19). Holy Spirit, come. In the name of Jesus, Amen.

Non-Hodgkin's (and Hodgkin's) Lymphoma Healing Prayer

Lord Jesus, I need a miracle in my lymphatic system. Please command it to stop producing too many white blood cells and abnormal lymphocytes. Holy Spirit, come. Remove from me the symptoms of belly pain, chest pain and anemia. I know that as my immune system wins out, the fever and chills will go. So will the night sweats and swollen lymph nodes as You heal my lymphatic system. Thank You for Your healing Word, Lord: "Is anyone among you sick? Let him call for the elders of the church, and let them pray over him, anointing him with oil in the name of the Lord. And the prayer of faith will save the one who is sick, and the Lord will raise him up. And if he has committed sins, he will be forgiven" (James 5:14–15). In the powerful name of Jesus, Amen.

Rabies Healing Prayer

Lord, this fever is proof that my body is fighting off infection after this bite from the rabies-infected animal. But You can reverse this curse and heal me. First, I rebuke the spirit of death and declare that I will live and be well again. Thank You in advance, God, for taking away the dizziness, delirium, hallucinations and mental confusion. Heal me of the nausea, appetite loss, vomiting and difficulty swallowing, and protect me from the other dangers such as seizures, muscle paralysis, sensitivity to light, dilated pupils, stiff neck and drooling. Cause my lymphatic system to drain this infection from my body quickly and completely. Steady my mind from all confusion, anxiety, irritability and aggression, and make me strong and calm again. Holy Spirit, come. I trust You. I am in Your care. "He who dwells in the shelter of the Most High will abide in the shadow of the Almighty. I will say to the LORD, 'My refuge and my fortress, my God, in whom I trust.' For he will deliver you from the snare of the fowler and from the deadly pestilence" (Psalm 91:1–3). In the healing name of Jesus I pray, Amen.

Staph Infection (Non-MRSA) Healing Prayer

Heavenly Father, this aggressive infection is trying to wreak havoc in my body, but since I know You are my Healer, I am running to You for help. Antibiotics can do so much, but they come with drawbacks, so I ask You to remove this infection from me and restore my health, commanding my lymphatic system to drain the staph infection entirely from my body. Thank You in advance for taking away the blisters and boils, rashes and redness, pus and abscesses, and all the other symptoms such as abdominal pain, diarrhea, nausea, vomiting, chills and fever. Holy Spirit, come. Protect me from this infection entering my bloodstream and threatening my life, and I also trust You to keep those around me safe from its contagion. My eyes are on You, God. "And many followed him, and he healed them all" (Matthew 12:15). In Jesus' name I pray, Amen.

25

Integumentary System

Skin, Hair, Nails, Sweat Glands

Declaration

I am ready to receive any needed healing for my integumentary system and then do whatever it takes to walk in divine health. I know that God does not make me sick, and I ask Him right now to show me the root of my condition, whether it be physical, emotional or spiritual. I am ready to pray the prayer of faith, reverse the curse and unleash the blessing. By God's grace, I will watch my words, maintain my miracle or wait on God's perfect timing for healing. Amen!

Integumentary System Blessing

Wrapping up our body system blessings is the system that wraps, conceals and protects every other system we have already blessed—the integumentary system. It is comprised of the skin (five layers of epidermis), **Integumentary System** nails, hair and sweat glands, and I speak not only the blessing of health over them, but the blessing of rejuvenation and youthfulness. I declare that your skin—your body's largest organ, which weighs about ten pounds—is disease-free, blemish-free and able to receive vitamin D from the sun's rays in moderation and remain cancer free. I speak to the condition of your hair, nails and sweat glands and declare them full of life and vibrancy. From the top of your head to the tip of your toes, I declare you to be healthy, happy and walking in divine health! Let it be done according to your faith and in the mighty name of Jesus!

Visit lauraharrissmith.com/blessings for the video blessing.

Your Integumentary System's A-list

Avoid dairy, sugar, alcohol, excess salt, fried food, caffeine, junk food

Add avocado, berries, eggs, bone broths, coconut oil; *exercise, saunas*

Allow vitamins A, B complex, C, D3, E, K; calcium, iron, fish oil, biotin, zinc

Apply helichrysum, myrrh, lavender, frankincense, ylang-ylang oils

Anoint with oil daily and pray needed healing prayers and body system blessings

Ask your doctor or health care provider before making regimen changes

Your Integumentary System's Favorite . . .

Breakfast: smoothie with ½ cup blueberries, cranberries and almond milk; 1 avocado, ½ lemon, stevia

Lunch: bone broth soup with tomatoes, red kidney beans; green salad with tomato, walnuts, egg

Dinner: salmon or chicken with olive oil, garlic; roasted broccoli and carrots with olive oil, pink salt

Snack: citrus fruits, almond butter, yam fries with cinnamon, walnuts, green tea, deviled eggs stuffed with mixed avocado and ranch, 70–80 percent cocoa organic dark chocolate

Testimony

"So, with age has come thinning hair, but I guess I am reversing that! I did two things: I started using Laura's Quiet Brain Shampoo and Conditioner, and then I started praying the integumentary system blessing over myself. My hair is actually getting thicker in my fifties!" ~Julie

After reading the blessings and prayers, send all testimonies large and small to healing@lauraharrissmith.com.

Integumentary System Healing Prayers

Acne Healing Prayer

God, my skin seems to have a mind of its own. Please calm the inflammation and help me through this embarrassing season. Remove the redness, tenderness, blackheads, bumps and pus-filled pimples. Should there be infection, please touch and heal that, too, and please mend any follicles that are plugged with oil and dead skin cells. Holy Spirit, come. Help me strictly abide by the wisdom on this chapter's A-list so that my skin might be its healthiest. Restore to me my baby-soft skin, and heal all scars, Jesus. I know You understand scars with great compassion. "You stretch out your hand to heal, and signs and wonders are performed through the name of Your holy servant Jesus" (Acts 4:30). In Jesus' name I pray, Amen.

Burns Healing Prayer

Jesus, please restore my skin from the damage caused by this injury. Whether from fire, chemicals, electricity, hot liquids or the sun itself, please heal these burns from all degrees of injury and make my skin like new. Lord, if this is life threatening, I first thank You for saving my life. Thank You for bringing me relief from the pain. Please even soothe whatever is going on that I cannot see beneath the skin. Holy Spirit, come. Heal all blisters, peeling, redness, sweating, flushing and swelling, and take discomfort far from me. This will no longer be true of me: "For my sides are filled with burning, and there is no soundness in my flesh" (Psalm 38:7). In Jesus' name, Amen.

Eczema (Atopic Dermatitis) and Xeroderma Healing Prayer

Father, please bring peace to my skin and cause the inflammation to cease. Remove every trace of rash, peeling, flakiness,

270

dryness and fissures. I pray, God, that no matter where on my body this condition is, You would replace the rough redness with my normal soft, supple flesh color. My skin will not itch, burn or interfere with my social life in any way. Holy Spirit, come. Help me abide by the A-list advice in this chapter and nourish my skin, head to toe. "My soul longs, yes, faints for the courts of the LORD; my heart and flesh sing for joy to the living God" (Psalm 84:2). I pray it in the mighty name of Jesus Christ, Amen.

Hair Thinning / Loss (Alopecia) Healing Prayer

Lord, this may seem insignificant to some people, but it is not to me . . . I do not want to lose my hair. Lord, I thank You for dealing with this and I ask You to reverse the hair loss, whether it is male or female pattern baldness (androgenetic alopecia) in which the hair thins on the top and crown of the head, or whether it is telogen effluvium, where hair falls out after a stressful experience. If it is prostaglandin D2 balding (since the lipid compound, prostaglandin, has been found on the scalps of balding men) then remind me to eat lots of berries, which lower those prostaglandin levels and can decrease hair loss. Holy Spirit, come. Nourish my entire integumentary system and replenish what has been lost. "Why, even the hairs of your head are all numbered. Fear not . . ." (Luke 12:7). In Jesus' name I pray, Amen.

Hand, Foot and Mouth Disease (HFMD) Healing Prayer

God, please heal my child [or me] of this painful virus. "From the sole of the foot even to the head, there is no soundness in it, but bruises and sores and raw wounds; they are not pressed out or bound up or softened with oil" (Isaiah 1:6). Let this not be said of us, O God, because we are turning to You. Holy Spirit, come. Remove the virus from the body entirely, along with the rash, blisters, peeling, red spots and canker sores. Replace dehydration with hydration, fatigue with strength, and irritability with joy.

271

May the HFMD's fever, sore throat and coughing never return. I ask it all in Your name, Jesus. Amen.

Hives (Urticaria) Healing Prayer

Father, please put an end to this misery. It feels impossible to get away from the discomfort, but I know You have a solution for me that brings healing. Remove from my system the irritant or allergen that has caused this reaction under and on my skin, and bring peace to the discomfort. Holy Spirit, come. Take away the raised, red or skin-colored welts, and cause the swelling to go down. I reach out to You for healing and declare that there will be no more flare-ups and no more itching. "They begged him to let the sick touch at least the fringe of his robe, and all who touched him were healed" (Matthew 14:36 NLT). In Your name, Lord, Amen.

Impetigo (School Sores) Healing Prayer

Lord, heal my child [or me] of this painful skin infection. Bring comfort and restoration to the sores forming around the nose and mouth, both those that are oozing and those that have already crusted over. Soothe the blisters and rash, and please bring relief from all itching. I ask You to contain this infection and prevent it from spreading to others, and I ask that Your healing would remove it from deep within so that there are no more flare-ups. Holy Spirit, come. Please heal this so completely that there is no scarring on the skin, and I thank You in advance for answering this prayer. "His flesh was restored like the flesh of a little child, and he was clean" (2 Kings 5:14). In Jesus' name I pray, Amen.

Melanomas and Carcinomas Healing Prayer

O Great Healer, I need a miracle in the pigment of my skin, for it has become cancerous. But I believe Your report, Lord, and my literal flesh cries out to You with praise for being its Healer: "My mouth shall speak the praise of the LORD; and let all flesh bless his holy name for ever and ever" (Psalm 145:21 KJV). Holy Spirit, come. Please cause this cancer to leave my body now, in the name of Jesus, and may all growths and moles shrink and disappear at Your command. My skin will no longer be susceptible to darkening and the regrowth of melanomas or basal cell carcinomas. Thank You in advance for restoring my skin to its original condition. In the healing name of Jesus Christ, Amen.

Nail Issues (Stippled, Ingrown, Hangnails, Beau's Lines, Fungus) Healing Prayer

Lord, I believe You care even about this tiny part of me . . . my nails. All twenty! Please bring healing to the issues that are causing me such discomfort, whether there be a problem with nail growth, a fungal infection, tearing or splitting. Heal the nail plates, the nail beds, the cuticles, the nail folds, the lunulae and the nail matrixes. May all twenty nails be long and strong and grow perfectly within the boundaries You have laid out for them. Holy Spirit, come. I thank You that I will not be ashamed of my hands or feet, and that I will not suffer pain or infection in any of them anymore in the name of Jesus. "The effectual fervent prayer of a righteous man availeth much" (James 5:16 KJV). In Jesus' mighty name, Amen.

Open Wounds Healing Prayer

Jesus, my skin is the barrier between the rest of me and the outside world, and it is meant to protect my body from infections, among other things. But that barrier has been broken, and this open wound is leaving me and my bones, muscles, nerves, tissue, arteries and tendons underneath vulnerable. I receive Your healing right now for this open break in my skin, whether it be from diabetic ulcers, pressure ulcers, surgical wounds, lacerations, puncture wounds, amputation wounds, etc. I say to it, "Close and heal now, in the name of Jesus." God, cause my lymphatic system to drain any infection quickly. Please restore my epidermis, dermis and subcutaneous layers, as if the wound had never happened. May any eschar and slough also be removed. Holy Spirit, come. I give You this pain and discomfort, and I trade it in for peace and restoration. "For I will restore health to you, and your wounds I will heal, declares the LORD" (Jeremiah 30:17). Thank You for being my Healer, Jesus. It is in Your name I pray, Amen.

Psoriasis Healing Prayer

Lord God, my immune system is causing my skin cells to reproduce too quickly and build up, forming these unsightly, itchy dry patches and scales, along with reddened skin. Lord, I know it's not leprosy, but some days it feels as though it is, and I need You to heal me. "Heal the sick, raise the dead, cleanse those who have leprosy, drive out demons. Freely you have received; freely give" (Matthew 10:8 NIV). I receive restoration to my skin right now in Your name, and I thank You that stress, cold temperatures and infections are no longer triggers for flare-ups for me. Heal the dry, flaky, peeling skin, as well as any fissures, bumps and thick patches. I also declare that I will not have joint stiffness, inflamed tendons or small dents in my nails. Finally, Lord, I choose joy and not depression. This psoriasis will not steal my social life, my outlook on life or my joy. Holy Spirit, come. I receive Your healing now in Jesus' name, Amen.

26

Mind, Mood and Miscellaneous Healing Prayers

Testimony

"I prayed all Laura's healing prayers and body system blessings over the course of a few days. For a few days prior to this, I had been really struggling with feeling blue and very sad. I had lots going on and was feeling overwhelmed with sadness and confusion. When I prayed the blessings over myself, I could feel an immediate lightening of my spirit. I felt hope and optimism for the first time in a while. The saying 'I felt a weight was lifted off'—well, yes, it did feel like that!" ~Janet

After reading the blessings and prayers, send all testimonies large and small to healing@lauraharrissmith.com.

Mind, Mood and Miscellaneous Healing Prayers

Addiction Healing Prayer

Jesus, it takes so much work to be an addict. I am done with the secrecy, the lying and the lack that comes with spending my money on the wrong things. Holy Spirit, come. Please reveal my past woundings to me, those things that are the root causes of why I am medicating myself. I rebuke and resist the unclean spirits of rejection, addiction and death. And whether my addiction is to a drug, an activity, a chemical, a thing or a person, I declare that nothing nor anyone will sit on the throne of my heart but You. I also ask You to bring me into a new circle of friends and influencers so that I might walk in the freedom You are bringing to me. "So if the Son sets you free, you will be free indeed" (John 8:36). In Your name, Jesus, Amen.

Anxiety Healing Prayer

Lord, I do not want to be anxious. I want my heart safely to trust in You all day, every day, and even at night. Jesus, help me see Your face when I begin to worry, because I know that Your eye is never off me and that You are always working things out for my good. I declare that my reactions and stress level will not be out of proportion to the impact of events, and that I will not be restless while I am waiting on situations to resolve. I resist the racing thoughts and tendency toward negativity. Holy Spirit, come. I choose peace over panic attacks. I choose trust and patience. I choose joy. I choose to do as Your Word directs, "casting all your anxieties on him, because he cares for you" (1 Peter 5:7). In Jesus' name, Amen.

Attention Deficit Disorders (ADD or ADHD) Healing Prayer

Heavenly Father, You have gotten my attention. I need help. I know You can help me focus and stay on task, not to mention do my work and be productive. I pray that You would take from me the forgetfulness, absent-mindedness, difficulty paying attention and short attention span. Replace those with concentration and a good memory. If there is ever hyperactivity, please rewire my brain right at that moment and guard me from the impulsivity, aggression, irritability, excitability and fidgeting. Help me also not to engage in repetitive behaviors, and, Lord, grace my mind to learn. Heal me from all learning disabilities, depression, boredom and mood swings. Holy Spirit, come. I will fix my thoughts on You. "Casting down imaginations, and every high thing that exalteth itself against the knowledge of God, and bringing into captivity every thought to the obedience of Christ" (2 Corinthians 10:5 KJV). It's in Your name I pray, Amen.

Bipolar Disorder (Manic Depression) Healing Prayer

God, I feel as if there are two of me. I'm told that bipolar disorder cannot be cured, but I know that You are the God of the impossible. The real me is full of joy. The real me has a happy, successful life. The real me chooses faith in You and knows that You will not disappoint me. That is the me who I choose to be. Holy Spirit, come. Please heal my brain of all chemical imbalances that cause the manic episodes, reduced need for sleep and a loss of touch with reality. Also, please balance my mind and body and guard me from the depressive tendencies, low energy, loss of motivation and disinterest in daily activities. I also vow to You, O God, that I will not take my life, should suicidal thoughts come. Those are not my thoughts. Those are not Your thoughts. They are thoughts from the enemy, and with Your help, I resist them and choose Your thoughts instead. "We have the mind of Christ" (1 Corinthians 2:16). In Jesus' name I pray, Amen.

Chromosome Disorders Healing Prayer

Jesus, I have learned that my child has a chromosomal abnormality, and my heart wants to be devastated. But my spirit knows You are in control, so I am choosing to trust You. There are testimonies of children who have been healed of Down syndrome, Lord, and I definitely believe You can do that. I also know You can heal Edwards syndrome, Patau syndrome, Turner's syndrome, Klinefelter syndrome, cri du chat syndrome, Prader-Willi syndrome, Tay-Sachs disease or cystic fibrosis [see the cystic fibrosis prayer in chapter 16]. So whether the disorder includes the 5th, 7th, 13th, 15th, 18th or 21st chromosome, I am asking You now to rewrite the DNA and let healing flow to my child. If this is a progressive healing, then show me how to parent my child through this process, and be with us through each twist and turn in the road. Holy Spirit, come. I know You have us on the path toward joy and purpose. "For nothing will be impossible with God" (Luke 1:37). In Jesus' name, Amen.

Demonic Possession / Oppression Healing Prayer for Deliverance

Lord Jesus, I want to be free. I feel bound by demonic forces that are controlling my life. But right now, I command any spirit that cannot say "Jesus is Lord" to leave me and never return. I ask Your forgiveness, Lord, for opening any door to this dark stronghold, and I welcome You to shine a spotlight into my heart and show me which decisions I have made that brought about this oppression. Holy Spirit, come. I welcome You into my heart and life in a new way right now and ask You to set me free. "The seventy-two returned with joy, saying, 'Lord, even the demons are subject to us in your name!' And he said to them, 'I saw Satan fall like lightning from heaven. Behold, I have given you authority to tread on serpents and scorpions, and over all the power of the enemy, and nothing shall hurt you. Nevertheless, do not rejoice in this, that the spirits are subject to you, but rejoice that your names are written in heaven'" (Luke 10:17–20). Fill me, Holy Spirit. In the name of my Deliverer, Jesus, Amen.

Depression (Including Clinical Depression) Healing Prayer

O Balm of Gilead, I need You to soothe my mind and pour out Your peace over my life. Please cure any abnormal activity in the neural circuits of my brain, and cause my mental health to be a reflection of Your mind and Your thoughts. Please remove any biological, psychological and relational sources of distress in my life. I declare that I will sleep well, eat well, focus well, communicate to those I love and not become isolated. My energy level will increase, and I will be able to fulfill my daily commitments, responsibilities and activities every day, in Jesus' name. "And the king said to me, 'Why is your face sad, seeing you are not sick? This is nothing but sadness of the heart'" (Nehemiah 2:2). Holy Spirit, come. Thank You for lifting sadness from me and replacing it with the oil of gladness. In Your name I pray, Lord. Amen.

Dyslexia Healing Prayer

Holy Spirit, come. Touch me cognitively and physically right now and do a miracle in how I perceive written words. Lord, I ask You to help me read better, learn better and comprehend better. I declare that I will no longer struggle with memorization, spelling, reading, speaking, learning or even thinking. My mind will be clear, my thoughts will be organized and my speech will have no impairment. Confusion will be far from me, and my mind will now be graced to do amazing things—things I never thought possible. "According to your faith be it done to you" (Matthew 9:29). In Your name and to Your glory, Jesus, Amen.

Fatigue (or Chronic Fatigue) Healing Prayer

Jesus, help me. I am tired of being tired. I am ready to feel Your wind at my back and have the stamina to live my life. I receive, right now, Your healing for my body. I refuse to remain exhausted, depressed, anxious, weak and achy all over. I declare that I am not a slave to depression, anxiety, confusion or a lack of focus. I will be sharp, alert, strong and healthy. I will thrive! Holy Spirit, come. I know You have heard my prayer and will restore me to the energy of my youth. "For I will satisfy the weary soul, and every languishing soul I will replenish" (Jeremiah 31:25). In Jesus' name, Amen.

Fever Healing Prayer

Father, the presence of infection has caused my body to work to fight it off, and that has caused my body temperature to increase. Lord, I know that fever is not a sickness that needs healing, but that it represents an internal struggle with something else that does, so I ask You to heal my body and free it from this struggle right now. I declare that my immune system is fighting for me, as You designed it to do. I thank You that as this illness leaves, the infection leaves and the fever leaves. With those must go the chills, sweating, muscle aches, appetite loss, dehydration, headaches and weakness. "Truly, truly, I say to you, whoever believes in me will also do the works that I do; and greater works than these will he do, because I am going to the Father" (John 14:12). Holy Spirit, come. In Jesus' healing name, Amen.

Insomnia Healing Prayer

Lord Jesus, I am in need of rest. My body must have rest to function well, heal and be strong. Holy Spirit, come. I ask You to quiet my brain as I lie down at night and cause me to enter into deep sleep. Your Word is like medicine, so I declare Psalm 23 over myself: "The LORD is my shepherd; I shall not want. He makes me lie down in green pastures. He leads me beside still waters. He restores my soul. He leads me in paths of righteousness for his name's sake. Even though I walk through the valley of the shadow of death, I will fear no evil, for you are with me; your rod and your staff, they comfort me. You prepare a table before me in the presence of my enemies; you anoint my head with oil; my cup overflows. Surely goodness and mercy shall follow me all the days of my life, and I shall dwell in the house of the LORD forever." I declare that I will go to sleep, stay asleep and be rested for my activities the next day, every day. In Jesus' name I pray it, Amen.

Note: Consider visiting quietbrainoil.com to watch the infomercial and hear people's testimonies of relief from insomnia and more through my essential oil blend, Quiet Brain.

Mental Illness Healing Prayer

Heavenly Father, Your Word says that "when the righteous cry for help, the LORD hears and delivers them out of all their troubles. The LORD is near to the brokenhearted and saves the crushed in spirit" (Psalm 34:17–18). Well, I am crying out to You for deliverance and for healing in my mind. Help me reach out to others when I need help, and remind me to reach out to You most of all. Whether this is depression, schizophrenia, PTSD, bipolar, dementia, ADD, ADHD, autism or another diagnosis, I declare that my mind is being healed right now in the name of Jesus. [See the healing prayers for autism and dementia in chapter 11 and for the rest in this chapter.] All chemical dysfunctions are being balanced in Your name, and my thoughts will line up with those thoughts You want me to have. Holy Spirit, come. I will not be riddled with anxiety or depression [see those healing prayers in this chapter], but instead, I choose trust and joy. In the name of Jesus, Amen.

Nightmares and Night Terrors Healing Prayer

Jesus, fear is trying to get a grip on me and cause me to worry and be anxious. You designed my body to rest and find deep sleep, not be tormented by nightmares and night terrors. I declare in Jesus' name that my bedroom is off-limits to the enemy and his torments. I declare that I will not be tormented by evil spirits while I am awake or asleep, because I am a Christ follower who loves and forgives others the way Christ loves and forgives me. Lord, if the images I have seen in this dream are details You are trying to give me so that I might pray and protect someone, then I thank You and consider it a warning dream and not a nightmare at all. I will be victorious. I will not be afraid, "for God gave us a spirit not of fear but of power and love and self-control" (2 Timothy 1:7). Holy Spirit, come. In Your name, Lord Jesus, Amen.

Post-Traumatic Stress Disorder (PTSD) Healing Prayer

Lord, I need help recovering from the emotional trauma I have been through. Not everyone understands it, but I know that You do. Holy Spirit, come. Please heal my mind and cause even my memories to be healed. I receive Your healing and believe it is washing over me right here, right now. Help me walk away from this situation with the wisdom and lessons it brought me, but without the pain and trauma. Help me forgive, and in appropriate cases, forget. Whether the trauma occurred years, months, weeks or days ago, I know that You can cleanse my spirit and soul of all flashbacks. I resist all nightmares, heightened reactions, self-destructive behaviors, insomnia and anxiety. I declare that I will not be depressed, feel guilty or isolate myself and detach from others, and I will not let this keep me from being in social settings that can bring me further healing, such as church or Christian support groups. I am unafraid of this happening again and will not let it cripple my future, my relationships or me. "In God, whose word I praise, in God I trust; I shall not be afraid. What can flesh do to me?" (Psalm 56:4). In Your healing name I pray, Jesus. Amen.

Schizophrenia Healing Prayer

Father, my mind needs clarity. It needs Your truth to invade it and differentiate for me what is real and what is not. Heal me physically, psychologically, emotionally and even genetically. Cause my brain chemistry to balance with perfection and think only that which edifies me and glorifies You. Lord, let this healing extend to my speech so that I might speak what is clear and organized, and so that I might not cause myself or anyone else harm. I resist all delusion, forgetfulness, amnesia, disorientation, disorder and a false sense of superiority. I will not be depressed, afraid, apathetic or moody. I will be calm, not angry; satisfied, not discontent; and peaceful, not anxious. Lord, thank You for showing me what is real. Thank You for healing me from false voices, hallucinations and especially any paranoia. Holy Spirit, come. "Do not be conformed to this world, but be transformed by the renewal of your mind, that by testing you may discern what is the will of God, what is good and acceptable and perfect" (Romans 12:2). In Jesus' name, Amen.

Sleep Apnea Healing Prayer

God, I need better sleep. Psalm 127:2 says of You that "he gives his beloved sleep" (NKJV). I am Your beloved, and I am Your child, so I am claiming this verse as part of my healing regimen. Show me the other steps You want me to take for better and deeper sleep, whether it be losing weight, making lifestyle changes or getting breathing assistance. I want to sleep more and snore less, and I am trusting You to heal me or guide me to those people who can help me. I declare that I will be well-rested and not struggle with daytime sleepiness, nightmares, dry mouth, headache or weight gain. I also speak over my emotions, that I will not be depressed, irritable or given to mood swings. Holy Spirit, come. You are my joy, my resting place, and my Healer. I pray it all in Jesus' name, Amen.

Speech Disorder (Lisp, Stuttering, Mute, etc.) Healing Prayer

Note: I used to have a speech disorder as a child, a horrible lisp that could not be hidden or missed. I am ever so grateful for my second-grade teacher, Mrs. Holly, who got me the speech therapy I needed, and for my encouraging parents—my first audience—who sat through my endless childhood skits, poetry readings and presentations that paved the way for what I am doing today.

Lord, I am ready to open my mouth and be confident in what I say and how I say it. No matter what form of speech impediment I have—whether it be an articulation disorder, a fluency disorder or a voice disorder—I ask You to touch my tongue, lips and entire mouth and cause it all to function as You have created mouths to function. Send me to the right teachers or therapists to help me, if that's what I need, and I thank You that You are also giving me new and important things to say. "Open your mouth wide, and I will fill it" (Psalm 81:10)." Holy Spirit, come. In Your name, Jesus, Amen.

Suicidal Thoughts Healing Prayer

O God, I want to live. But I want to really live and be happy and healthy. I resist the lie that says I will be better off just coming to be with You. If You wanted me with You now, then You would have brought me home already, but You are leaving me on this earth for a purpose. What is that purpose, Lord? Show me a glimpse of my future so that I might trust You and hold on. Lord, show me which Christian friend I need to call right now who will walk through this with me and remind me of Your will for my life.

I declare that I will not always struggle with depression, anxiety, bipolar, schizophrenia [see the healing prayers for all of these in this chapter] or any other mental disorder. Holy Spirit, come. My mind is healed, and my spirit is hopeful for the future, "For you have delivered my soul from death, my eyes from tears, my feet from stumbling" (Psalm 116:8). In Your name, O Lord, Amen.

Tourette's Syndrome (TS) Healing Prayer

Jesus, help me overcome this tormenting force called Tourette's syndrome. Touch my brain—physically and mentally—and heal it of all the symptoms and the many tics. Calm my eyes from unwanted blinking, my shoulders from unwanted shrugging, my muscles from unwanted jerking, my throat from unwanted clearings and my body from uncontrollable repetitive movements. Lord, most of all guard my mouth. I will no longer succumb to an unclean, foul spirit's whispers to me, nor will I speak the script it writes for me. I am God's mouthpiece, not Satan's, and my speech will reflect that. "A Prayer of one afflicted, when he is faint and pours out his complaint before the LORD. Hear my prayer, O LORD; let my cry come to you! Do not hide your face from me in the day of my distress! Incline your ear to me; answer me speedily in the day when I call!" (Psalm 102:1–2). Holy Spirit, come. In Your healing name I pray, Jesus. Amen.

Tumors Healing Prayer

Heavenly Father, my heart is trying not to be afraid. Whether malignant or benign, I don't like the sound of the fact that I have a tumor, and I certainly don't like the prospect of surgery or radiation. So I am turning to You first for healing. Holy Spirit, come. Shrink this tumor entirely, by the power of Your touch.

Note: Place your hand on the tumor now, or have someone else do it.

Lord, cause this abnormal growth of tissue to dissolve right now and to disappear entirely. Command the physiological process that has caused this uncontrollable and abnormal division of cells to reverse and stop this cycle now, in Jesus' name. Lord, if You prefer a progressive healing for me with the help of remedies, then lead me to them. I know You hear this prayer and will answer. "The eyes of the LORD are on the righteous, and his ears are attentive to their cry" (Psalm 34:15 NIV). In Jesus' mighty name I pray, Amen.

Weight Management (Overweight/Underweight) Healing Prayer

Lord, I know You like me just as I am, but I don't like how I look. Right now, I choose to see myself as You see me and get Your strategy for a new and improved body. Whether I need weight gain or weight loss, You know how to unlock my body's metabolism and bring balance. Holy Spirit, come. Lead me to the right lifestyle changes that bring me the results I need, because the desire of my heart is to be healthy. I declare that I will do whatever it takes to get healthy, including exercise, better food choices and more rest. And I will not do it through eating disorders [see the eating disorders prayer in chapter 17] but the right way, paying special attention to any organs that need better nourishment and health. And until I get to my goals, I declare that I will like myself and resist the insecurity that the enemy wishes for me. I am secure in You. "I will heal them and reveal to them abundance of prosperity and security" (Jeremiah 33:6). In Your name, Jesus, Amen.

Get Well, Stay Well

Now that you have had all 15 of your body systems blessed and have been given access to more than 200 healing prayers for just about whatever ails you, you may still need some help in getting your healing prayers answered in the form of improved health. So, in this third part of the book, you will learn how to troubleshoot stubborn illnesses and better understand what might be standing in the way of your healing or miracle. I have also included a closing benediction in which I pray for and bless any part of you that, for whatever reason, has escaped your attention in parts one and two—body, mind or spirit.

After the benediction, you will find the book's very convenient infirmity index. Since the healing prayers are organized within the individual body systems (as opposed to one long, alphabetized prayer list) the infirmity index is a tool you can use that will allow you to locate quickly the healing prayer you need, right when you need it. Less time searching means more time praying and faster healing. The title of this book is not *Get Well*, but *Get Well Soon*, and it is my earnest goal to help you do just that.

27

Troubleshooting Stubborn Illnesses

There are times when you pray fervently and do all that is biblically required of you to position yourself for a miracle, and it still does not come. What you do in the early stages of that reality is very important to ensure that you do not fall into unbelief about your situation ever changing. If you do fall into unbelief, the situation certainly may not change. I am believing something better for you, however. I am believing in faith for immediate miracles to take place whenever you need to turn to one of the 200-plus healing prayers inside this book, or even after you just read one of the 15 body system blessings.

Yet I also know from experience that sometimes God both desires and allows a different healing path. A path of patience. I talked about this path in chapter 10, and about the importance of keeping an eternal perspective when it does not appear that your healing is going to manifest. It is easy to get a finger pointed at you, accusing you of having little faith. I have experienced it. Or maybe someone judges that some hidden sin is preventing the manifestation of your miracle. Or maybe you are the one doing the pointing and judging. Let that never be said of us. To behave that way is to behave as Job's friends did, and we saw what happened to them. God rebuked them (see Job 42:7–9).

What we must do is simple. Not always easy, but simple. We must look with spiritual eyes at our broken physical situation. We *must* seek God about the roadblock. What looks like a stubborn illness might not be an illness at all. Rather, it could be a spiritual battle that is merely manifesting itself bodily. If you have done everything you can do in the natural—nutrition, medicine, rest—and your problem does not go away, then it may have its roots in the spirit realm. The good news about that, however, is that once you determine what the spiritual battle is, you can get "God's prescription" for the situation, deal with the root in the spirit realm (through prayer and deliverance), and then watch your body respond to the process. It *will* respond. It is just another perfect picture of a "by process" healing. It is like incremental breakthrough, but make no mistake, breakthrough comes.

When you find yourself in a situation where a stubborn illness just will not let go, and you have done everything medically and nutritionally possible to get well, then take some time to step back, put on your spirit lenses and ask yourself one of the following four questions:

1. *Am I battling a demonic harasser, as Paul did with his 2 Corinthians 12 thorn in the flesh?* If the answer to this is yes, then as we said in chapter 3, God is "entrusting" to you a demonic messenger to defeat through prayer, because He has found you equipped to do so (and this was my journey). If the answer is no, then go on to question 2.

2. *Am I dealing with a generational curse?* If so, return to chapter 6 and review how to break generational curses,

and then pray and ask God to reveal any of those curses in your family, along with a prayer strategy for how to reverse them. You can be the repairer of the breach in your family! If you do not feel this is your issue, then continue on to question 3.

3. *Am I not watching my words, and therefore undermining the miracle God wants to do?* If this is the problem, then revisit chapter 7 for a refresher on the vocabulary of waiting. If this is not your issue, then go on to question 4.

4. *Has God chosen a healing for me and not a miracle?* If so, what could He be wanting to do in you—body, mind and spirit—through a "by process" healing? Revisit chapter 9 so that you can get excited about God's design for your breakthrough.

After leaving no stone unturned in helping you get well soon and stay well for life, I am still painfully aware that some people never heal, and that even more people graduate to heaven "too early," leaving behind loved ones who must then reconcile their faith with their new reality. For those of you who are still pursuing healing for your body, or even healing for your heart, I want to be vulnerable and open a window into my soul by sharing a story with you. On my nightstand are two pictures that are the first things I see each morning. One is a Scripture with Jesus' words from Mark 16:18 about how believers will lay hands on the sick and they will recover. The other is a picture of my best friend, Sheila, on whom I once laid my hands, yet she did not recover. So I ask you, does not this contradiction perfectly depict our journey of faith in this fallen world? Do our losses mean the Bible is not true? Do they reveal that Jesus did not mean what He said? Do they mean the supernatural is not for today?

No. What Sheila would tell you if she were here today—and in fact, what she told me on her deathbed—is that there are hidden variables in every man or woman's journey of pursuing the Creator for healing, none of which involve God wavering. He is not a man, that He should lie. We are mere mortals, and do. Daily we fall short of the glory of God, and yet daily His Word remains true. The secret, therefore, to avoiding the loss of one's faith when a loved one does not recover after much prayer is to continue to believe every inch of God's Word and trust that you just did not know everything about the situation, the way you think you did.

The alternative? To rearrange your theology to match your experience, and then to dilute the Good News. Friend, we must preach the Gospel, not our experience. There is always another explanation besides God or His Word being fallible, and we have covered some of them in these pages: generational curses, personal sin, unwise health choices and even just the sick person's fatigue in the final stretch.

Sheila told me at the very end that the more she pressed into Jesus for healing, the more she just wanted to go live with Him. And trust me, it was not that she did not love her family.

I could not accept this decision of Sheila's, and I flew back and forth three thousand miles round trip to see her more than once and beg her not to give up. But I have seen it happen with other giants in the faith, who just decide that they want to go home and then do so *very* quickly, despite how hard the rest of us are praying.

So . . . I leave these two framed paradoxical pictures side by side on my nightstand to remind myself every morning that in my full-time ministry of bringing health and healing to others—including you—I will never have all the answers. Just like you, I walk by faith and not by sight. But I have decided that if I err, then I will always err on the side of faith, for God's Word will never fail.

"This God—his way is perfect; the word of the LORD proves true" (2 Samuel 22:31).

28

Benediction

My friend, you have just successfully:

1. Decided just how well you want to be
2. Taken inventory of your health
3. Acknowledged that God did not make you sick
4. Discovered the root of your condition
5. Learned how to pray the prayer of faith
6. Prepared yourself for the unleashing of the blessing and the reversing of the curse
7. Learned how to watch your words
8. Discovered how to maintain your miracle
9. Understood the difference between a healing and a miracle
10. Prepared yourself to meet (and love) the new you

Those are the ten steps you have taken, and now we have added one more that you just accomplished successfully:

11. Learned to troubleshoot stubborn illnesses

You have also been challenged to get moving and add exercise to your daily and weekly routine, asking God for the best strategy for your situation and schedule. And I am happy to report that now, at the end of writing this book, I have put in 90.1 miles on this exercise bike desk. (I tracked fewer miles in part two because it is difficult to pedal and pray at the same time.) I learned that climbing to the top of Mount Everest is only a 5.5-mile challenge, so I figure that I have conquered Mount Everest more than 16 times while writing this book for you. I also learned that more people die descending Mount Everest than they do ascending it. Therein lies a lesson for you about retaining everything you have learned in this book during your mountaintop experiences while reading it. Don't stumble on the way down by forgetting them.

Also now at your disposal is an arsenal of 200-plus healing prayers, whether you read all of them upfront or save them for a rainy day. Certainly, part two is the part that will keep on giving, so keep *Get Well Soon* near your medicine cabinet or church altar for decades to come.

Finally, I hope you enjoyed and will continue to employ the 15 body system blessings for your entire body daily, and I hope you will take advantage of the videos I made of speaking the blessings over you myself at lauraharrissmith.com/blessings.

Now I want to leave you with a closing blessing. *Benediction* is a word I absolutely love. As an informal definition, *bene* means "good," and *diction* means "word," as in *dictionary*. So what I am doing through this benediction is leaving you with a "good word." I have written a poem for you that invokes and invites health to each of your 15 body systems, starting with your nervous system and going in the order they appeared in this book, all the way to your integumentary system, and also through the mind, mood and miscellaneous areas. I leave you now with this good word, and I pray that it becomes your new reality as you walk in divine health all the days of your life:

May your head be full of blessing
from brain to mind to moods
May your eyes be sharp and focused
May your mouth desire God's foods

May the messengers in your bloodstream
dispatch their news on cue
Each timed hormonal signal
that somehow makes *you* you

May your blood fulfill its missions
May your vessels take it there
May your heart beat with precision
May it never know despair

May your lungs expand with vigor
and not once be short of breath
May your appetites be bridled,
choosing life and never death

May your body use each nutrient
distribute then digest
May your thirst be quenched and satisfied
disposing of the rest

May your loins inherit legacy
or your womb deliver life
May the oneness of the Church and Christ
unite husband and wife

May your frame be strong and sturdy
Bone and sinew in its place
May you conquer every mountain
and finish every race

May you be immune to sickness
and to poverty and rage
May you oversee and guard your health
so it guards you in old age

May your skin be thick but supple
despite what life unveils
May your head not lose a single hair
when fighting tooth and nail

May the Holy Spirit fill you
when your life you must defend
May you never fail to get well soon
and stay well 'til the end.

Infirmity Index

Laura Harris Smith is a certified nutritional counselor with a master's degree in Original Medicine. But before all of that, she was just a farmer's daughter with a love for colorful food, and a pastor's granddaughter with a heart to see others prosper spiritually. The bestselling author and her husband, Chris, are the founding co-pastors of Eastgate Creative Christian Fellowship in Nashville, Tennessee, where they specialize in helping people get healthy—body, mind and spirit—believing it is the only path to wholeness.

In television for more than fifty years (since she was three), Laura is the executive producer and host of *theTHREE*, her body, mind and spirit show that airs every day of the week all over the world. Laura is also the inventor of Quiet Brain® Essential Oil Blend and its growing product line, including Quiet Brain candles, shampoo, conditioner, inhalers and diffusers.

Laura is the author of more than twenty books and e-books, including the bestselling *The 30-Day Faith Detox: Renew Your Mind, Cleanse Your Body, Heal Your Spirit* (Chosen, 2016), *The Healthy Living Handbook: Simple, Everyday Habits for Your Body, Mind and Spirit* (Chosen, 2017) and *Seeing the Voice of God: What God is Telling You through Dreams & Visions* (Chosen, 2014).

Married for 35 years, Chris and Laura have six adult children: Jessica, Julian, Jhason, Jeorgi, Jude and Jenesis. They are all homeschooled, all writers and all gifted communicators. With half of them grown and married, "the grandmuffins" now far outnumber the kids.

Invite Laura to speak: booking@lauraharrissmith.com
Official website: lauraharrissmith.com
Television: theTHREE.tv
Quiet Brain: quietbrainoil.com
Chris and Laura's Nashville church: eastgateccf.com
Facebook: facebook.com/LauraHarrisSmithPage/
Twitter: @LauraHSmith

More from Laura Harris Smith

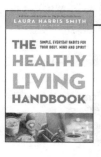

Accessible, practical and grounded in real life, *The Healthy Living Handbook* is full of simple, everyday ways to live a truly healthy life—body, mind and spirit. These easy-to-implement lifestyle tips will not only bring the peace, rest, energy, connection and clarity you've been longing for, but help you to live better in every area of life.

The Healthy Living Handbook

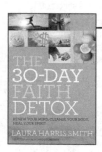

Invisible faith toxins can cause symptoms that affect our entire being—mind, body and spirit. In this one-month detox, expert Laura Harris Smith uncovers thirty faith toxins and promotes biblical healing of the whole person through prayer, Scripture and simple recipes. Refresh and refuel yourself spiritually, mentally and physically with this practical guide.

The 30-Day Faith Detox

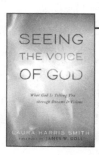

With absorbing insight, *Seeing the Voice of God* demystifies nighttime dreams and daytime visions, revealing the science behind the supernatural and giving you a biblical foundation for making sense of what you see. Includes a comprehensive Dream Symbols Dictionary with over 1,000 biblical definitions.

Seeing the Voice of God

✔Chosen

Stay up to date on your favorite books and authors with our free e-newsletters. Sign up today at chosenbooks.com.

 facebook.com/chosenbooks

 @chosen_books

@Chosen_Books